# Sober Living

## A Work Book to Overcome Your Addiction

by

## Paul "Pablo" Noddings

**This book is dedicated to <u>You</u>, with Love!**

**Please claim this book by writing your details below:**

Your Name:_____

Cell Phone Number: _____

Drug of Choice: _____

Emergency Contact Name: _____

Emergency Contact Number: _____

# Prologue

Your dilemma is a life-and-death struggle!

Do you stay in your familiar misery

of your uncontrollable drug and alcohol use?

Or do you take the chance at a better life

and the possibility of finding love?

# Table of Contents

# My Story

My name is Pablo, and I am a recovering alcoholic and drug addict. Today, I am clean and sober, and I have been since January 6, 2015.

I grew up on the coast in the 1970s. My parents were loving, and we went to the beach often, where I enjoyed swimming in the sea. By the age of ten, I had my own surfboard and I identified as a "surfer." I still surf and I still identify as a surfer. Surfing is a healthy activity—an outdoor lifestyle—a sport that brings you closer to nature and in rhythm with the universe.

The use of alcohol and marijuana was common within my circle of surfing friends. As a young surfer, I looked up to the older surfers. Most of them drank beer and smoked weed. As I got older and became a better surfer, I was included in the group of older boys, and soon I was drinking beer and smoking weed too.

This started out as innocent experimentation. In my opinion, it was part of the development of a teenage boy into a young man. My problems came much further down the line. I surfed throughout my time in college and I continued to indulge in drinking beer and smoking weed. I tried smoking cigarettes, but I didn't like them; they tasted foul to me. However, I enjoyed smoking weed because it made me feel relaxed.

After college, I was a hard worker with a demanding job and after work, I would play hard by surfing, playing rugby, and hitting the gym. When I got home at night, I drank beer and smoked weed in order to "relax" because stress was always present. Most people have loads of stress, and I am no exception. I had education stress, relationship stress, self-employment stress and financial stress. I thought I allowed the stress to run off me well, but like a dam slowly filling with water, my stress level kept building. The same is probably true for most other people.

My problems with alcohol and marijuana were growing, and I knew it for at least ten years before I could stop using them. I was trapped in the cycle of drinking "a few more beers" and having "another smoke of weed" until I would get so loaded that I was fully baked. I do not think this is a big deal if I did this once in six months but my problem was that I did this every night for thirty-three years, and there was an escalation in how much I indulged in drinking and smoking. I tried to stop smoking weed many times, but I was never successful for more than a few days.

I would get "loaded" in the evenings and stay home because I knew there was no chance of attracting anyone who interested me while I was "bleeding from the eyes" and unable to talk without slurring my words. I was single and I had never been married, but I wanted to find a loving partner. I'd had relationships over the years, but they seemed to end abruptly. I would spend six months trying to figure out what went wrong before I would try again with someone new.

The loneliness was crushing! On several occasions, I held my head in my hands and cried because I was so lonely; I couldn't bear to live with myself! I felt I was a prisoner to beer and weed, but I couldn't stop. I was stuck in a vicious cycle of addiction with no way out. I had slid into addiction just like every other addict. The details of your story will be different to mine, but the slide into addiction is common to all of us.

Then, I had an unexpected, life-changing event. I went surfing at a surf break called "Four Mile," which is four miles up the north coast from Santa Cruz, California, where I had lived for fifteen years. I had been surfing Four Mile as my main break for many years. That day, I didn't walk along the base of the cliff to enter the water from the rocks as I normally did. Instead, I used the rip current to take me into the middle of the bay and I paddled across the bay towards the surf break. While I was in the deep water in the middle of the bay, I saw the dorsal fin of a large shark rise to the surface of the water and come straight at me. I blinked several times to make sure I was not imagining things and I realized I was in a seriously dangerous situation! The shark was swimming abnormally fast, and it was coming straight at me!

I was certain this would be my last day alive. My number had been called by "the man upstairs." I would die in a pool of blood and bubbles, and no one would know until my surfboard washed up onto the beach hours later.

The shark was swimming fast—straight at me—and I could see a fountain of water peeling off each side of its dorsal fin as it approached. Time slowed down and my life flashed before me, including all the things I had not done but wanted to do. I felt a deep fear, but I managed to remain calm enough to make the decision to face the shark head-on and fight it!

Being eaten alive by a shark is a primal fear, and my sensors became hyper-alert. I could see tiny black spots on the camouflaged mottled gray dorsal fin, which was producing a barreling wave peeling off each side of its leading edge.

I expected the shark's head to rise out of the water with its mouth open and bite down on me. I positioned myself to thrust my surfboard into its mouth, but the shark submerged inches from the front of my surfboard and passed underneath me. I turned my head to face it and waited a second. When it did not re-appear, I started paddling as fast as I could. While paddling, I looked back one time, expecting to see the dorsal fin following me. I frantically searched the sea for the shark but looking back scared me so much that I chose to focus on paddling with long, powerful strokes.

It took me at least two minutes to get to safety. My adrenaline was so high that I was unable to sleep for two nights, I couldn't even lie down for more than a few seconds. I was so amped up that I had to walk around the small town of Santa Cruz in the middle of the night for two nights in a row. For three days and two nights, I was wide awake and happy to be alive.

This traumatic event was the catalyst that made me realize what was truly important to me. When my life flashed before my eyes, drinking beer and smoking weed were unimportant. To me, leading a meaningful life with as much love as possible was what mattered most.

I was unable to stop drinking and smoking immediately after, however this event propelled me toward recovery from addiction. After I became serious about my recovery, I relapsed four or five times before I was successful in overcoming my addiction. With each relapse, I learned more about what triggered me and I gained an understanding of my personal problems that manifested themselves as addiction. I realized that for me alcohol and weed went together like bacon and eggs. I knew that I had to quit both of them if I was going to quit either of them.

A major asset that helped me in overcoming my addiction was Alcoholics Anonymous and I will forever be grateful to AA. The first time I went to an AA meeting, I introduced myself by saying, "My name is Pablo, I am an alcoholic and an addict." I immediately felt a weight lift off my shoulders. I had admitted to a room of peers that I had a problem, and the problem suddenly felt more manageable because of my admission. I did not find the twelve-step program helpful in my recovery, although I believe that many people have found this program to be helpful. For me, it was simply admitting to others that I have problems that manifest as addiction which are too big for me to handle on my own and knowing that there is a place to go where there are many other people who admitted the same. The public admission was a major step forward for me. It has become increasingly clear to me that this type of honesty is extremely important to recovery and a meaningful life.

I planned my detox date, and I struggled hard to not use for the first few days. I had to constantly tell myself "NO!" The first week was incredibly difficult, and the first month was almost as difficult. After three months of being sober, I felt that I had too much to lose to relapse. It was around the six-month mark that I felt much more in control. I felt myself moving toward my new life rather than constantly telling myself "no" to my old life.

I sometimes get cravings to use alcohol or marijuana, but they don't last long. My thoughts of using are replaced with knowledge of the chaos and misery drugs and alcohol would bring into my life.

I own a four-unit rental property in Santa Cruz, California. As these units became available for new occupants, I filled them with people who want to live in a sober living environment. I live on this property myself, and I manage it with a small team of my clients. This has given me a large amount of experience with people who are recovering from addiction. This experience, along with my own recovery, are the foundations of this book.

# Introduction

This book primarily addresses people recovering from addiction to alcohol, heroin, stimulants and benzodiazepines because these are the drugs of choice of most of my clients. The principles in this book can be used to assist in recovery from addiction to any drug, as well as addictions to gambling, gaming, food, work, sex, or social media. Even "normal people" can benefit from the principles in this book.

My opinions are presented with love, and they are intended to help you in your recovery. You may not agree with all my opinions, but that is not necessary for you to benefit from this book. I encourage you to use everything you find helpful and reject the rest.

The subjects covered in this book are roughly in order of importance, with the most important subjects being covered first. You can read this book quickly using the table of contents and the chapter outlines as summaries. I encourage you to write in this book as you read it and I encourage you to refer back to this book often.

The path to recovery from addiction is **not** a secret! It is easy for me to show you the path to recovery, but this does not make it an easy path for you to travel. A summary of the path to recovery from addiction is that you start by admitting to yourself that you have an addiction, then you take specific physical actions for at least six months and during this process you take control of your mind. This path has been traveled by millions of people before you and you can travel this path too. The most important ingredients for your success are your motivation and your persistence to achieve sobriety, even if you relapse.

In fact most people relapse. An all-too-common cause of death for addicts is a relapse overdose, which happens by using the same quantity and strength of the illicit substance you were using before you quit. Your body's tolerance for your drug of choice is reduced during your clean time, so a relapse can easily cause a critical overdose. If you start using again, please use a small quantity and immediately plan another attempt to quit. Don't give up on recovery just because you relapse—be persistent! Try as many times as it takes. You will relapse less and less frequently until you escape addiction for good.

Recovery from addiction is difficult but staying in addiction is worse! You have suffered enough that you are looking for help. Your situation has gotten so bad that there is no alternative for you but change. Waving a feather at your recovery from addiction is unlikely to succeed, you need to smash your addiction with a ten-pound hammer! You need as many odds in your favor as possible to achieve sobriety. This book will help you to do that.

Recovery is worth your effort!

Good luck and enjoy the ride as best you can.

# Part 1: Prepare Now

# 1.1: Your Addiction

The first step to recovering from your addiction is to admit your addiction to yourself! Fully recognizing your addiction is important because most addicts spend years convincing themselves, and others, that they don't have a problem with drugs or alcohol.

The process of overcoming addiction has to start with your sincere acknowledgement that an addiction exists.

Even if other people can see your problem from a mile away, some addicts will remain blind to their addiction and blame their "bad luck" on anything other than their obvious drug or alcohol problem. Some addicts will lose their marriage, their children, their job, their home, all their money and *still* refuse to admit that they have an addiction problem! They might get incarcerated for a DUI or other drug offense and continue to use drugs in prison, where it is dangerous and expensive to do so, and they may blame everything except their addiction for the situations they find themselves in.

What is your "rock bottom?" How far do you have to fall before you will admit that you have an addiction and that it is the root cause of your problems? The earlier you recognize your addiction, the better.

Some addicts choose to run away from their problems rather than simply to admit them. Do not do this! It is better to face your problems head-on and fight them. The only thing you accomplish in trying to escape your problems is to cause more problems. Perhaps you move to a new city, find a new lover, or try a new drug and that becomes your excuse as to why now is not the time to deal with your addiction.

There are approximately two million people in the U.S. system of federal prisons, local jails, and detention centers, and 75% of these people will spend more than five years in prison. The Federal Bureau of Prisons reports that approximately 46% of all inmates are in prison for drug and alcohol offenses, making it by far the most common reason for incarceration (see www.bop.gov/about/statistics ). What percentage of these people admit to themselves that they have a problem with addiction?

An addict has three choices for their future: incarceration, death, or recovery. Are you going to continue in your addiction until you find yourself in jail or end up dead? Or are you going to admit you have a problem with addiction and start your journey to recovery?

# 1.2: Your Responsibility

Most people who slide into addiction have suffered trauma—emotional trauma, physical trauma and generational trauma. Although trauma and its effect on us are very real, you should not define your life by the trauma you have suffered. If you adopt a victim mentality, it becomes easier for your trauma to manifest as addiction and lead you down the dark path of addiction.

You have the ability to anticipate the consequences of your actions so you are largely responsible for the situation you find yourself in. This is good news because if you take responsibility for your addiction, you can take back control of your life and you will have a better mindset to overcome your addiction.

To break the cycle of addiction, admit your addiction and take responsibility for it. Take responsibility for yourself and the situation you find yourself in. If you google the word "responsibility," you will see that the word means to have to deal with something or have control over someone. If you take to heart your responsibility for your recovery, your chances of success are much higher because you will have removed the victim mentality.

Seeing yourself as a victim is to see yourself as too weak and too helpless to make changes. If you take responsibility for the position you find yourself in, you will have the power to choose differently.

Imagine yourself as an alpha character, the person who takes charge, the decision maker and the leader. This character type may be foreign to you but try to adopt this character type when dealing with taking responsibility for the position that you find yourself in. Seeing yourself as responsible for your position will put you on a solid path of recovery, and you will need to keep this mentality of strength because you are going to face many challenges on the road ahead.

# 1.3: Your Motivation

The most critical ingredient for your success in recovering from addiction is how strongly motivated you are to quit drugs and alcohol.

The only person who can make this happen is YOU, the addict! You can't rely on someone else to do this for you, not your parents, not a government program, nor some imaginary super-hero. They cannot save you. _You must save yourself!_

Addicts often feel powerless to control their addiction. But admitting your addiction, taking responsibility for your addiction, and understanding your motivation to quit your addiction will start the process of regaining your power.

Once you have been using drugs and alcohol heavily for more than ten years, you get very little pleasure from it. Initially, using drugs and alcohol provides you with an escape, but after many years, it becomes your prison, impinging on your freedom to develop a meaningful life. You have become trapped in your addiction and you need to break out of its grip.

Recovery from your addiction should be the primary responsibility that you whole-heartedly accept as the driving force of your life.

Addiction has defined your life for too long, now let recovery define your life. I encourage you to make a conscious decision to make your recovery from addiction the primary motivation of your life. Decide for yourself to bear this burden. Embrace this struggle. Make recovery the central pillar of your existence.

This type of strong, willful, conscious motivation is required to break free from addiction. The stronger your determination to break out of addiction, the better your chances of achieving sobriety.

Understanding the reasons why you use drugs or alcohol and investigating why you want to quit using drugs and alcohol will help you to be successful. Sex and power are two primary motivations for human behavior. Humans are hard-wired to provide an answer to the question of their sex drive, whether that drive is large, small, or weird and humans are hard-wired to gather as much power as they can. Power is the control of scarce resources such as food, money, or attention. When you investigate the reasons why you are using drugs or alcohol, consider how sex and power play a role in your addiction.

The list of questions below is an exercise to help you better understand your addiction and your motivation to recover from addiction. This is not a substitute for a professional counselor who can help you to explore this subject in much more depth. These questions are simply a conversation starter on the subject of your motivation to quit drugs and alcohol.

Engage with this book. Now is the time to get a pen and write in this book!

**Direction: Write down your answers to these questions.**

1. What age were you when you started using drugs or alcohol?

   _____

2. What is your drug of choice?

   _____

3. What are the secondary drugs that you use?

   _____

   _____

4. What was your progression of drug and alcohol use?

   _____

   _____

   _____

5. What is your daily/weekly consumption?

   _____

   _____

   _____

6.   How much does your daily / weekly consumption cost?

_____

_____

_____


7.   How do you get the money to afford your addiction?

_____

_____

_____


8.   Why do you want to stop using drugs and alcohol?

_____

_____

_____

_____

_____

_____

_____

# 1.4: Keep a Journal

Keeping a journal, or diary, is an inexpensive, yet life-changing tool that you can use to help you overcome your addiction. You can use an old-fashioned notebook, or you can use a computer or phone app. Use whatever works best for you. This simple tool can help your recovery tremendously! I highly recommend it, so much so that at the end of this book, you'll find some pages included for you to use as a starting point for your journal.

Please start journaling while you are still using. Write in your journal every day, listing all the drugs and alcohol you use, including the amount and cost. Note whether you could control your cravings and how you felt every time you used.

Keeping a journal is having a written dialogue with yourself. The act of recording your thoughts is a therapeutic exercise. Some people find it beneficial to have a written record of their thoughts so they can review them at a later date. In my experience, I seldom revisit my old journal entries. It is mostly the act of writing in my journal that I find helpful because it forces me to organize my thoughts and to ask myself the simple question "What are my thoughts?"

Each day, write in your journal about something you have done well. Focus on what you did that was positive or felt like an accomplishment. Even if it is something small, take the time to compliment yourself. This is a healthy exercise, and it is helpful to your recovery, as you will start to see yourself in a more positive light.

When you stop using and begin detox, journal about your feelings and your pain. Use your journal to express yourself and let out your unfiltered emotions.

In early recovery, write in your journal about your cravings and how you have had to tell yourself "no" repeatedly. Keep written notes about how you overcame your cravings. This can be helpful in controlling yourself in the future.

Even if you relapse, keep up with your journal because it will give you insight into the reasons for your relapse. Keeping a journal will increase your understanding of your underlying problems that manifest themselves as addictive behavior, and this understanding will help you to be more successful.

## 1.5: Routines and Rituals

It is very important to build healthy routines and rituals that will assist you in getting through your days without using drugs and alcohol. A ritual is simply a routine that is done with a greater sense of purpose or in a more intensional manner.

The more routines you can keep up, the better. Write down your routines. The more detailed these written routines are, the easier it will be to follow them with little deviation. You can use your routines to keep yourself busy, which helps during periods of cravings when your inner voice is chatting excessively and incorrectly guiding you to use drugs and alcohol.

If you are constantly thinking about using drugs or alcohol, use your routines to get through the next few minutes or the next few hours without using. In the first weeks of not using, you are going to rely heavily on your routines. You may need them for six months or more before your routines become so practiced that you don't have to consciously think about them.

Most addicts live in chaos and do not have healthy routines to fall back on. I have suggested a few simple routines as a starting point so that you can write down your own set of routines.

**Direction: Please alter my routines below to fit your schedule:**

1.5.1: Wake-Up Routine

| | |
|---|---|
| 6:00 a.m. | Wake up |
| 6:15 a.m. | Get out of bed |
| 6:30 a.m. | Make bed |
| 6:40 a.m. | Make coffee |
| 6:50 a.m. | Make a list of actions to do |
| 7:00 a.m. | Start with the most important action |

1.5.2: Daily Routine

| | |
|---|---|
| 6:00 a.m. | Wake up with an alarm |
| 7:00 a.m. | To-do list |
| 7:30 a.m | Walk |
| 8:00 a.m. | Work |
| 10:00 a.m. | Eat breakfast |
| 10:30 a.m. | Work |
| 4:00 p.m. | Eat dinner |
| 4:30 a.m. | Work |
| 7:00 p.m. | Walk |
| 9:00 p.m. | Go to bed |

1.5.3 Weekly Routine

| | |
|---|---|
| Monday | Work |
| Tuesday | Work |
| Wednesday | Work |
| Thursday | Work |
| Friday | Work |
| Saturday | Clean home |
| Sunday | Practice personal care |

This is a particularly simple weekly routine, but it shows the basic concept of getting out to work five days a week and setting aside the other two days for taking care of cleaning your home and practicing personal care. Create your own home cleaning routines and personal care routines.

There are many other routines that may suit you better. I encourage you to write them down in this book and expand on them over time so that you improve your chances of recovery from addiction by having as many routines as possible to rely on when you are saying "no" to cravings to use drugs or alcohol.

**Direction: Please write down your routines below:**

_____

_____

_____

_____

_____

_____

_____

_____

_____

_____

_____

_____

_____

# 1.6: Church and Religion

In this chapter, I discuss formal church and religion, not spirituality, which I cover later in chapter 4.5.

Wikipedia states approximately 84% of people on planet Earth are religious, with Christianity, Islam, Hinduism, and Buddhism being the four largest religions. There are 7.8 billion people on planet Earth in the year 2022 which means that 6 billion, 550 million of these people identify as religious. This is a very large group of people. Most of these people belong to the dominant religion of the geographic region into which they were born.

The different religions around the world have far more in common with each other than differences. Most religions have a set of rules of behavior that participants are expected to follow and these rules are very similar across all religions. Most religions teach that there is a power higher than yourself, and most religions have an explanation of life after death. They also tend to have distinct architecture for their churches and a holy book that they reference.

In my opinion, there is little difference between the different Gods of the various religions because much of the teachings of the religions have very similar content. If you are dissatisfied with the main four religions, you might investigate the Pagan religion. Pagans believe that nature itself is God, they embrace ancient practices and are unstructured by comparison to the main four religions.

Don't outright reject religion on the basis of some small detail. There are some conflicting details between the major religions, so not all religions can be 100% correct about every point of detail. It is unlikely that you'll find a religion where you whole-heartedly believe every single detail contained within its doctrine.

You should never argue with someone over religion; rather, you should keep the conversation agreeable and save your thoughts until you can privately investigate any details with which you might disagree. If your disagreeable detail creates an untenable situation, quietly move to another religion.

What matters most is that a large group of people are involved with religion and there are major benefits to you to be part of this group. You should strengthen your relationships with other people in religious organizations for the benefits of connection to community and access to resources. You should choose a religion that is convenient for your location and appeals to you in some way. You should investigate multiple religious organizations and see what each has to offer. It may be beneficial for you to have a relationship with more than one religious organization in your area. Over time, you will gravitate toward the organization that fits your needs best.

Start the process of strengthening your relationships with churches before you quit drugs and alcohol. It will help your recovery to have these relationships, and it will give you a better chance at staying sober. Many big churches have a recovery ministry for the purpose of helping addicts through recovery, and some even offer financial support for sober housing. These organizations provide you the opportunity for friendships with people outside your old circle of "friends" who are still using drugs.

To be successful at quitting drugs and alcohol, you need to use everything you can to your advantage and increase your odds of recovering from your addiction. Religious organizations offer community and this is helpful for your recovery from addiction.

I encourage you to be open to the possibility of a religious epiphany while you are developing your relationships with religious organizations; however, do not make this your goal. If an epiphany occurs at some point along the way, this is a bonus for which you should be grateful.

**Direction:** Write the names of Churches and Religions that you will associate with:

_____

_____

_____

_____

_____

_____

# 1.7: Psychological Help

I am not a licensed therapist, psychologist, or drug counselor, and I recommend the use of these professionals. Many counselors charge for their services on a sliding scale. Meaning, your cost is based according to what you are able to pay. If you don't have much money, you can seek a free consultation with counselors who are working toward getting their license. These counselors are typically younger, and they can be valuable to have as part of your support team. Patients and counselors in the U.S. can connect at www.psychologytoday.com. Most other countries have a similar resource.

I recommend that you connect with mental health professionals before you quit drugs or alcohol so that you improve your chances of successfully recovering when your "get clean date" arrives and you stop using. Seek out drug counselors, psychologists, and family therapists. It is better to rely on professionals like these for support instead of family or friends who may unintentionally cause you more harm with poor advice. Also, your family and friends may be part of the reason why you started down the rabbit hole of addiction in the first place.

An internet search for mental health professionals in your area is likely to produce many results. Find several that looks like a match for you and call them to make an appointment and start the process of working with them. The important part is to make contact and get the process started. It can take weeks or months to get onto the schedule of a mental health professional so it is important to start the process now!

Mental health professionals can help you in ways you may not have known you needed help. Most people with mental health problems are unaware of their problems. You may have an undiagnosed psychiatric condition and you may be using illicit drugs to compensate for this condition without realizing it. Common examples include using cocaine as a pick-me-up when you feel depressed or habitually using benzodiazepines when you feel anxious. If underlying mental health conditions are being disguised by drug use, it is essential to discover what these issues are as part of your recovery process. Conversely, heavy drug use may have caused a psychiatric condition that you did not have before and you may not be aware that you have this condition now.

The most challenging problems that I face running a sober home are mental health clients who present themselves as addicts in recovery. Clients who have mental health issues are often unaware of the issue and are un-diagnosed, not medicated and not seeing a mental health professional.

If you have been diagnosed with a mental health condition, it is essential that you take any medications prescribed to you as directed by your doctor. It is also essential that you stay in communication with your medical support team to maintain your mental health care throughout your recovery.

Depression is a common mental health condition, and SSRI drugs (selective serotonin re-uptake inhibitors) are frequently prescribed to treat it. Depression is a feeling of alienation from society, a separation from community, and a feeling of being alone. This concept is called "duality," which means it's "you versus the world". Anything that promotes "non-duality," or a connection with others, is likely to help. Mental health professionals are your go-to experts who help you overcome depression and other mental health conditions.

Another common mental health condition within the addiction recovery community is bipolar disorder. This is when a person oscillates between two extremes in mood—depressed and manic (hyperactive). Sometimes the person is not consciously aware of the shifts in their mental state. Many addicts with bipolar disorder stop taking their prescribed medications because they prefer one mood over the other, or they may decide on their own that they are no longer bi-polar and they stop taking their medication. Professional help and medications have proven very effective at treating bi-polar conditions. Those with bipolar disorder must take their medications as prescribed while they are attempting to recover from an addiction to illicit drugs.

Other psychiatric conditions that are less common including schizophrenia and sociopath disorders. Schizophrenia is a chronic (long-term) mental disorder that affects less than one percent of the U.S. population. Symptoms of schizophrenia can include delusions, hallucinations, disorganized speech, trouble with thinking, angry outbursts, facial contortions and lack of motivation. "Sociopath" is a psychiatric condition for a person with an anti-social personality disorder manifesting itself in apathy for the suffering of others. A psychopath is basically a more extreme sociopath. Although these conditions are rare, there is a greater chance of encountering these mental health conditions within the addict community because mental health and drug addiction are closely linked.

There are two areas where you must provide your own psychological self-help as you prepare for your recovery from addiction. The first is getting good quality sleep, covered more in chapter 3.6.4 below. The second is getting music that you find relaxing. Relaxing music will calm your mind and improve your mood control. This subject is deep, and many experts are doing research into psycho-acoustic medicine, vibration therapy, binaural beats, cell frequencies, and human energy. These deep subjects offer hope for the future, but for your purpose at this time, relaxing music can be obtained by a transistor radio or one of the many music streaming services on the Internet.

It is important to be aware that "normal" people who may not otherwise have a mental health issue can still experience psychological deterioration with age. This can be genetic or caused by a brain tumor. These cases are rare, but they should not be ignored.

Having a psychiatric professional, or two, on your recovery team is a good idea! It can be done at a low cost because most psychiatric professionals charge for their services on a sliding scale, allowing people with very little money to receive services at low costs.

**Direction:** Write down the names and contact details of mental health professionals that you plan to contact. Call them today because it can take several weeks or months to get onto their schedule:

_____

_____

_____

_____

_____

_____

_____

_____

# 1.8: Medical Help

I am not a doctor and I do not offer medical advice. I recommend the use of qualified doctors, and I encourage you to have a good relationship with a doctor as part of your preparation for your recovery from addiction.

It is extremely helpful to pre-plan your medical support resources before your "get clean date" arrives. Make a list of the nearest Doctors on Duty offices, your county's medical clinics and any local hospitals. Even if you do not have insurance, most hospitals will not turn you away if you are in critical, life-threatening danger. You should know where the nearest hospital is and what medical resources are available to you before you start your journey of recovery.

It is best for you to look for Doctors who specialize in assisting addicts to recover from addiction, but if this is not available to you, work with any qualified doctor.

**Direction:** Write down the name and contact details of medical professionals that you plan to contact:

_____

_____

_____

_____

_____

_____

_____

_____

## 1.9: Medically Assisted Treatments - MAT's

Medical doctors can prescribe medication which assist addicts with detoxification and staying off illicit drugs in the long term. The recovery community calls this medically assisted treatment (MAT). I have seen more people succeed in their recovery by using MAT options than I have seen without them. Using MAT options means that you have a medical professional as part of your recovery team and that is already a good start.

A general practitioner Doctor who has no experience in MAT's or the off-label use of the drugs listed below is unlikely to feel comfortable prescribing them to a patient who is looking for help in overcoming addiction but if this is the only Doctor you have access to, work with them. You will be in a better position if you can find a Doctor who specializes in assisting people recovering from illicit drug use.

Pre-planning the use of one or more of these drugs can help you through the most difficult periods of detox, and they can be helpful in quitting drugs and alcohol permanently.

The most common MAT drugs are listed below to help you to become familiarized with this category of medicine. Use this list as a reference. These prescribed medications are intended as a conversation starter with your medical professional.

The nine medications listed below are legal in California with a prescription from a qualified medical professional. I recommend that you start a conversation on this topic with any medical professional whom you have access to.

# 1.9.1 Pharmaceutical MAT's:

### 1.9.1.1: Antabuse - Alcohol

The drug Antabuse blocks an enzyme in the liver that breaks down alcohol. If a patient drinks alcohol while on this drug, they become violently ill. The theory is that the alcoholic won't want to drink again due to the unpleasantness of their experience. However, this can be circumvented if the patient stops taking the medication before they begin drinking again, in which case, the relapse would have to be pre-planned.

## 1.9.1.2: Naltrexone or Vivitrol - Alcohol and Opiates

Naltrexone was approved by the FDA in 1994, and Vivitrol was introduced to the market in 2010. Vivitrol is a once-per-month injection of the opioid agonist naltrexone, which is slowly released into the bloodstream over the course of the month. This will completely block the effects of any opiates.

Interestingly, it has also been used, sometimes in an oral form, to treat alcoholism, as it removes any pleasurable sensations from alcohol. Many alcoholics lose interest in alcohol after just one drink, and that is life changing for them!

The potential danger from this drug is that a person can end up consuming far too much alcohol in pursuit of a "high" that never materializes, which can cause alcohol poisoning or an overdose.

## 1.91.3: Methadone - Opiates

Methadone was introduced to the market in the 1970s. It is a synthetic substitute for heroin that has the endorsement of the U.S. government, with methadone clinics set up across the country in an attempt to provide a safer alternative to heroin.

Methadone is a pure agonist, like heroin, which allows an addict to use a large dose of methadone to get a "high." Additionally, addicts can use other opiates on top of methadone.

It is important to be aware that methadone is a synthetic opioid medication that causes physical dependence. Ideally, the user should lower their methadone dose to zero over a period of approximately one year, although some users simply swop heroin for methadone and are on methadone for many years. There are people who believe that it is harder to get off methadone than it is to get off heroin.

Methadone can cause side effects such as constipation and weight gain. There are other drawbacks, mostly caused by the policies governing the ways methadone is provided to patients. Patients must go to a methadone clinic to receive their daily dosage until they build up a level of trust with the clinician over a lengthy period of time. After that, patients are given a "take-home dose." In theory, this is a reasonable model; however, maintaining a work or school schedule can be difficult, as patients must visit the clinic every day to keep a steady dose of methadone in their systems. Being seen near methadone clinics can reduce the recovering addicts anonymity and many of those who hang around methadone clinics are not committed to recovery or are still using drugs in conjunction with their methadone. This makes the environment risky for someone who is trying to abstain from all illicit drugs because illicit drugs may be readily available in the car park of the methadone clinic.

## 1.9.1.4: Suboxone or Subutex - Opiates

Suboxone and Subutex are both trade names for buprenorphine, which is a mixed agonist-antagonist that discourages relapse by blocking the effects of the opiate high, and providing a ceiling effect. Suboxone and Subutex also contains a small dose of Naloxone to discourage attempts at abuse.

Suboxone and Subutex are available via prescription from a doctor who has undergone a brief training session and certification on this drug. Suboxone and Subutex are available from a regular pharmacy, which makes it less stigmatizing for patients. Once a patient's dose stabilizes, it is virtually impossible for a third party to detect it use from the outward appearances of the patient.

Suboxone and Subutex are intended for long term use. Opiate addicts with a history of multiple relapses should consider Suboxone and Subutex as an MAT option to improve their chances of breaking their cycle of relapse and to achieve recovery from addiction permanently.

## 1.9.1.5: Clonidine - Opiates and General

Clonidine is in a class of medications called centrally acting alpha-agonist hypotensive agents. It treats high blood pressure by decreasing your heart rate and relaxing the blood vessels so that blood can flow more easily through the body. Clonidine will reduce your blood pressure, which can help to reduce opioid withdrawals. Clonidine extended-release tablets may treat ADHD by affecting the part of the brain that controls attention and impulsivity.

### 1.9.1.6: Trazodone - Anti-depressant and Sleep

Trazodone is in a class of medications called serotonin modulators, which work by increasing serotonin—a natural substance in the brain that helps maintain mental balance. Trazodone is an antidepressant that is often used to help normalize sleeping patterns which are disrupted by the withdrawal of many illicit drugs.

### 1.9.1.7: Gabapentin - Seizures and Anxiety

Gabapentin is in a class of medications called anticonvulsants, and it treats seizures by decreasing abnormal excitement in the brain. It also relieves the pain of post-herpetic neuralgia (PHN), which is a burning, stabbing pain that may last for months or years after an attack of shingles.

Gabapentin was originally used to treat fibromyalgia and nerve pain but has since been prescribed off-label for many conditions. Gabapentin also reduces the severity of opioid withdrawals and may have a calming, anti-anxiety effect.

### 1.9.1.8: Klonopin - Anxiety

Klonopin is a benzodiazepine drug. It lacks many of the dangers of other benzos, such as Xanax, but it can still cause dependency and it can be abused. Klonopin is used for patients coming off a very long-term benzo addiction and can be a stabilizing alternative that is overall less dangerous.

### 1.9.1.9: Clonazepam - Seizures

Clonazepam is an anticonvulsant or anti-epileptic drug used to prevent and control seizures; it is also used to treat panic attacks. Clonazepam works by calming your brain and nerves.

## 1.9.1.10: Ketamine - Anesthesia with Off-Label Uses

Ketamine is a medication primarily used for induction and maintenance of anesthesia in humans and animals during surgery. It is a general, short-acting anesthetic with hallucinogenic effects that induces dissociative anesthesia—a trance-like state providing pain relief and sedation. This drug can used as an illicit drug to cause dissociative psychedelic effects and it has been used to facilitate sexual assault crimes.

Ketamine is legal with a prescription in the State of California, and it is sometimes prescribed off-label to treat depression, anxiety, chronic pain, PTSD, OCD, alcohol, and substance dependencies. Normally, this is done in a clinical setting with constant supervision. Doctors who prescribe ketamine this way usually specialize in medically-assisted treatment for recovering addicts and alcoholics.

**Direction:** Write down the names of the pharmacehtical MAT's that interest you the most?

_____

_____

_____

_____

_____

_____

_____

_____

_____

# 1.9.2: Plant Based MAT's:

The next seven medically-assisted treatments are plant-based treatments. The first four of these are currently illegal in California, but they are legal in Mexico, Canada, Jamaica, and elsewhere.

Plant Based MAT's have become more popular because they offer an alternative to addicts who have failed with pharmaceutical MAT's and because a segment of the population have more confidence in remedies offered by nature.

### 1.9.2.1: Psilocybin (Magic) Mushrooms - Psychedelic

John Hopkins University is a leader in studying the benefits of psilocybin mushrooms on patients dealing with anxiety, depression, PTSD, and recovery from addiction. There have been small-scale studies showing promising results in assisting long-term smokers to quit tobacco permanently. Similar results have been achieved assisting alcoholics and heroin addicts to quit. With results like these, it appears that psilocybin mushrooms can positively contribute to modern society due to their ability to help alleviate mental health issues.

Psilocybin mushroom treatments should be guided by a trained clinician and have consideration to set and setting. Set means there should be a pre-written plan of intent for the experience and setting means there should be a physical environment that is comfortable, relaxed, and safe. There should be a qualified "trip sitter" to attend to the needs of the patient. Music and a comfortable place to lie down is desirable, and your schedule should be free for the day so you do not become anxious during your session about other commitments. The following day should also be a low stress day to facilitate your re-integration to your normal life after an experience that could have a significant impact on you.

Psilocybin mushrooms are on the path to legalization by several States. The State of Oregon has legalized the use of psilocybin mushrooms. The cities of Denver, Colorado and Oakland and Santa Cruz, California have passed laws decriminalizing the use of psilocybin mushrooms.

## 1.9.2.2: Ibogaine - Psychedelic

Ibogaine is a psychedelic drug derived from the root of a bush native to West Africa. Its therapeutic effects are not well-known, and it is illegal in the USA. It has a remarkable and almost immediate impact on eliminating opioid withdrawal symptoms. Although the physical symptoms of opiate withdrawal can last anywhere from one to three weeks, if a dose of ibogaine is taken just as the patient is entering the beginning stage of withdrawal, it seems to halt the effects and block them for the duration of a normal withdrawal period, as well as for a couple of months afterwards.

Some people have described Ibogaine as an "off switch" for heroin addiction and say the dreamlike nature of the psychedelic experience provides a therapeutic space to help work through some of the personal issues or traumas that might have been keeping the addict stuck in their addiction.

Numerous clinics in Mexico, Canada, and other countries offer this treatment to those desperate for alternatives, and many of the testimonials are positive. For most people, this treatment option will cost approximately ten thousand dollars when you include the cost of travel, accommodations, food, and payment to the medical clinic. It is illegal in the USA, where it is classified as a schedule I drug, which means that the Food and Drug Administration (FDA) considers this compound to have no known medical benefits.

Ibogaine is the strongest plant-derived psychedelic drug and the "trip" this drug induces is often intense and long lasting (12-36 hours). Ibogaine is considered male and is referred to as the "Stern Father" for the candid way it reveals the truth of the user's past. Ibogaine induces an introspective experience that can scare users.

The following five treatments originated in South America, specifically the Amazon jungle region. This is an area with interesting biodiversity that is receiving more academic study from western institutions.

## 1.9.2.3: Ayahuasca - Di-Methyl-Tryptamine (DMT)

Ayahuasca is a brew made from the leaves of the *Psychotria viridis* shrub along with the stalks of the *Banisteriopsis caapi* vine and includes the psychoactive ingredient di-methyl-tryptamine (DMT). DMT provides a spiritual experience, including dreamlike hallucinations, during which the patient is conscious.

Advocates of Ayahuasca believe that ingesting additional DMT resets our neurochemistry and mood by stabilizing low dopamine or high serotonin.

Ayahuasca works quickly, going straight to the root of your problems and cornering you to face your problems head-on. Advocates of Ayahuasca believe that it can achieve in one day what talk therapy may take ten years to accomplish.

This drug can take you to the depths of your psyche and cause intense personal revelations that can help you in your recovery from addiction. Ayahuasca can also take you to the nether regions of the multiverse and expand your consciousness.

At high doses, the experience can be extremely intense and can cause vomiting, diarrhea, or purging. The duration of the intense part of an Ayahuasca trip is approximately four hours, and the positive long-term effects can last for months or years. Ayahuasca is considered female and will guide the user with a mother's love.

The compound DMT is already within each of us in our spinal fluid, brain, eyes, and possibly our Pineal gland, the gland which is referred to as our "Third Eye" that allows us to feel an inner connection to other people and the "vibe" of our environment.

The Pineal gland is symbolized by the pine cone because it looks similar to a tiny pine cone and there are examples of this symbolism in ancient stone carvings as well as in the Vatican City today. This singular gland is housed between the two hemispheres of the brain and it is connected to the same part of the brain that our eyes are connected to. The Pineal gland is activated by darkness and it is believed to control circadian rhythm and influence dreams.

When the shark that I encountered at Four-Mile was swimming straight at me, my life flashed before my eyes in less than one second. It was as if a video tape of my life was played at hyper speed within the eye of my mind. This was a very real experience for me and I remember it clearly ten years later. I wonder what role my Pineal gland played?

## 1.9.2.4: Huachuma - Psychedelic

Huachuma is ingested as either a dried powder or a bitter, viscous tea made from the most potent parts of a San Pedro cactus. It is mainly comprised of mescaline and it was originally used by the indigenous people of Peru and Bolivia. Nowadays, the San Pedro cactus can be found in many climates and it grows well in California.

The process of turning the San Pedro cactus into Huachuma involves chopping the cactus into chucks, boiling it for hours and reducing it to a concentrated liquid or powder containing mescaline. Mescaline is illegal in California. Texas is the only state where peyote harvesting is legal. Peyote also contains mescaline and the preparation of peyotes into mescaline can only be done legally by a person who is registered with the State of Texas.

Proponents of Huachuma claim the benefits to be healing a broken heart, improving a sense of connection with people and nature, and treating alcoholism.

The final three MATs discussed below are legal in California.

## 1.9.2.5: Rapéh - Tobacco

Rapéh (pronounced 'ha-peh' in English) is pure tobacco, also called mapacho, that is indigenous to the Amazonian jungle and a sacred shamanic snuff medicine.

Rapéh can be purchased online. It is administered in the nasal cavity by using a pipe called a Tepi, made from bamboo, wood, or bone. It can be self-administered using a V-shaped self-applicator pipe called a Kuripe, which connects the mouth to the nostrils.

The benefits of Rapéh are increased clarity, reduced anxiety, and the removal of energy blockages. It is common to cry, purge, sweat, or otherwise release energies that were previous blocked, and Rapéh lowers blood pressure and calms the nervous system. It can relieve anxiety and provide a sense of trust and safety.

This product should be used infrequently because, like most tobacco products, it can be habit-forming. Rapéh is often used in conjunction with other indigenous ceremonies.

## 1.9.2.6: Sananga - Eye Drop

Sananga is an eye-drop with a painful sting and can be used by itself or as a precursor to Ayahuasca ceremonies. It can be purchased on the Internet for approximately $45 a bottle.

Sananga is made from the roots and bark of the *Tabernaemontana undulata* shrub, a "milkwood" species in the family *Apocynaceae*, and comes directly from the Amazon jungle.

This sacred, potent medicine is used for healing physical and spiritual ailments by clearing the mind and gaining new perception. Sananga is healing for inner sight, intuitive guidance, and opening of the third eye.

## 1.9.2.7: Kambo - Peptides

Kambo is legal in California and can be purchased online as a sticky paste attached to a small, paddle-like stick from which it can be scrapped off and used.

Kambo is made from the secretions of the skin of a green frog that lives in the trees of the Amazon Rainforest. This frog is the *Phyllomedusa bicolor* and the more common name for this frog is "giant tree frog."

This medicine contains over 100 different chemical constituents, which results in a profound opportunity for detoxing. The most famous of the alkaloids in Kambo is a series of peptides that trigger temporary hyperactivity in the immune system. While working with Kambo can be a very intense experience, the journey is short, not psychotropic, and offers a long list of therapeutic benefits.

Kambo's magical peptides are just beginning to receive the study and reverence they deserve. They are known to help with a massive list of ailments, including chronic pain, hormonal imbalances, lymphatic blockages, immunity deficiencies and other diseases.

Kambo is applied through superficial burns that pierce the first layer of the skin. This gives the medicine immediate access to the body through the lymphatic system. Kambo is known as "Warrior Medicine" because it helps us to tap into our resilient core and shows us how capable we are of handling discomfort.

The heart of a Kambo experience involves a massive purge. This purge helps to remove toxicity, energetic blockages, and stuck emotions. Kambo is an extremely strong physical experience, so it is essential to work with a trained practitioner. Kambo can raise and lower blood pressure rapidly, so losing consciousness is not uncommon, making it more crucial to have someone watching over you throughout the process.

The benefits of Kambo include alleviating depression and anxiety. Kambo is also effective with acute and chronic pain of all kinds. It is a massive anti-inflammatory and goes straight to the source of injuries and traumas. Another benefit is a boost to the immune system. The peptides in Kambo can create an experience of "super immunity." It is fortifying and supports the body to fight off harmful viruses, bacteria, and illnesses.

**Direction:** Write down the names of the Plant Based MAT's which interest you the most?

_____

_____

_____

_____

_____

_____

_____

_____

_____

_____

In summary of MATs, I recommend that you work with medical professionals to develop a regiment of medically-assisted treatments. Find a doctor who specializes in MATs and has experience with patients recovering from addiction.

Your team of medical professionals should include shamans, wellness coaches, and personal healers if you are interested in plant-based medicines.

Your preparation to quit using illicit drugs is an important part of the overall recovery process.

**Direction:** Please write down your Quit Plan below.

# Quit Plan:

1. What is your planned "get clean date"? _____

2. Where will you live in the first week/month of detox? _____

3. Where will you live after your initial detox? _____

4. Names/phone numbers of the people you have informed about your Quit Plan?

_____

_____

_____

5. What Churches and Religions will you associate with?_____

_____

_____

_____

6. What mental health professionals are part of your recovery team? _____

_____

_____

_____

7. What medical professionals are part of your recovery team? _____

_____

_____

_____

8. What Pharmaceutical MAT's will you use? _____

_____

_____

_____

9. What Plant Based MAT's will you use? _____

_____

_____

_____

**Direction:** Please write down your Quit Plan below.

# Quit Plan:

1. What is your planned "get clean date"? _____

2. Where will you live in the first week/month of detox? _____

3. Where will you live after your initial detox? _____

4. Names/phone numbers of the people you have informed about your Quit Plan?

_____

_____

_____

5. What Churches and Religions will you associate with?_____

_____

_____

_____

6. What mental health professionals are part of your recovery team? _____

_____

_____

_____

7. What medical professionals are part of your recovery team? _____

_____

_____

_____

8. What Pharmaceutical MAT's will you use? _____

_____

_____

_____

9. What Plant Based MAT's will you use? _____

_____

_____

_____

**Direction:** Please write down your Quit Plan below.

# Quit Plan:

1. What is your planned "get clean date"? _____

2. Where will you live in the first week/month of detox? _____

3. Where will you live after your initial detox? _____

4. Names/phone numbers of the people you have informed about your Quit Plan?

_____

_____

_____

5. What Churches and Religions will you associate with?_____

_____

_____

_____

6. What mental health professionals are part of your recovery team? _____

_____

_____

_____

7. What medical professionals are part of your recovery team? _____

_____

_____

_____

8. What Pharmaceutical MAT's will you use? _____

_____

_____

_____

9. What Plant Based MAT's will you use? _____

_____

_____

_____

# Part 2: Stop, STOP, #STOP!

Are you scared to quit drugs and alcohol because the detox is too hard?

Be honest with yourself about your life, where you live, how you get money, and what you represent. Take control of your response to your addiction and stop using drugs and alcohol.

This chapter will focus on getting you through the early stages of quitting your addiction.

## 2.1: Stop Using and Detoxify

Write the Quit Plan with your "get clean date" in the previous chapter. Choose this date in advance and plan for your period of detoxification. Some illicit drugs should have a tapering-off period so as not to send your body into withdrawal shock.

There are addiction treatment centers that specialize in helping people detox. I recommend that you take advantage of these facilities if possible. Private detox centers are expensive, costing approximately $1,000 per day, and most will require you to commit to being a patient for one to four weeks. Premium health insurance plans will cover some or all of these costs, but most addicts don't have health insurance.

If your health insurance plan will not cover your detox or you do not have health insurance, you must look for an opening in a government detox program. Many of these programs do not have the capacity to meet the demand for their services, which means that a hard-core addict has to stay addicted until an opening becomes available, or the addict has to detox on their own.

Some recovering addicts rent a room in a house for a week for the specific purpose of getting off the streets and trying to stay clean. Some addicts try to stop using and detox in the same living environment where they were using. This could be their car, a home, a sidewalk, or a clump of trees. Depending on your level of addiction, this can be dangerous. There may be better options for you.

I recommend showing your dedication to recovery by camping out in front of a detox center and other non-violent methods of communication that show how serious you are about overcoming addiction. If you are persistent, you will find an opening in a detox program somewhere. And when you get your chance, you must take it without hesitation.

Whether you are in a treatment center to kick-start your recovery or you are doing it on your own, when your planned "get clean date" arrives, you need to STOP!

Recovery from drug addiction means you STOP USING!

Put yourself on a tight leash and control yourself. In the first days of quitting, you will need to be brutal with yourself. Say "NO" every single time you think about using.

Detox is not easy for anyone, especially for those who have been using for a long time. You should go into it knowing it will not be easy, so you won't be surprised when you struggle. If you have done the preparation that I have discussed in the previous chapter, it will help you to get through your toughest times.

Even if you can only stop using for a few hours or a few days, this is better than not trying to stop at all. Your first day will be hard but days two through seven will be even harder. Your first week is likely to be as hard as any week and your first month is likely to be your hardest month. This is good news because your hardest time is likely to be at the beginning. By month three, controlling your cravings will be a little easier but your will still be struggling with cravings and self control. After six months of sobriety, I felt attracted towards my new life rather than saying "No" to my old life but each person is different and recovering from your addiction will take you as long as it takes.

Keep writing in your diary. You will learn more about your use of drugs and alcohol and your ability to recover from addiction.

The following section lists several helpful principles to follow once your "get clean date" arrives and you are in the early stages of recovery.

## 2.2: Do Not Stress – Live Here and Now

Keep your stress levels low. Don't panic. Don't stress out.

Stress will increase your chances of a relapse. Take stress seriously and do all you can to avoid it. Try to avoid doing any physical or mental activities that will cause you stress. Family relationships, sexual relationships, money, and travel are major sources of stress for most people. An addict in early recovery should avoid these completely.

Most people get stressed by the scenarios they create in their minds more than the actual reality of the moments they experience. Our thoughts run ahead of our reality with many scary what-if scenarios that cause us to suffer from situations that don't exist. Our minds chatter with scary scenarios that are unhelpful to an addict on a journey to recovery. Practice being in the moment and recognize the "power of now" and try to quiet the chatter of your mind!

Live in your immediate environment rather than the various frightening scenarios your mind conjures up. At this very moment, you are likely safe and relatively comfortable. Focus on your breathing and the feeling of the air entering your lungs and giving you the gift of life. You should not let your mind run wild with scary scenarios that are unlikely to become reality. This is not helpful to you.

Living in the moment and stringing those moments together to live without drugs or alcohol for a few seconds at a time and then a few minutes at a time. This will get you through your initial periods of cravings. In the first few days of quitting, just live moment to moment. Expect this to be difficult because every addict finds the first few weeks to be very difficult! Eventually, you will be able to "live one day at a time" without drugs and alcohol, but it may take weeks or months to get there without serious cravings to use every minute of every day. If you find yourself constantly thinking about using, this is normal, but you must say, "NO!"

Use the routines we discussed earlier to help you get through the worst of it and busy yourself with other tasks to divert your attention away from using drugs and alcohol. Routines will give you tasks to do and keep you busy so that you focus on something other than your cravings. It is good to TAKE ACTION. Go for a walk, do an activity, do anything other than use drugs and alcohol. Taking action will reduce your stress.

To keep your stress levels as low as possible, keep your life simple! Eat, sleep, and follow your healthy routines.

## 2.3: Do Not Drink Alcohol

In early recovery, do not consume any alcohol whatsoever, even if alcohol is not your drug of choice. Alcohol is the primary gateway drug that leads people to use other drugs.

Drinking alcohol will weaken your resolve to stay off your drug of choice. After you have had "a few drinks," you are more likely to use your drug of choice. A person with an addiction to meth or heroin has very little chance of saying "no" to meth or heroin once they have a "buzz" from alcohol.

You've probably heard the saying "if you hang around a barbershop, soon you will have a haircut." Similarly, if you go to bars, soon you will have a drink. If you are in recovery from addiction, do not go to bars or other places where alcohol is served. If you go to events where drugs or alcohol are present, it is likely you will end up using, so it is best to not go to these events at all.

In early recovery, do not see the people you were previously seeing regularly. Do not go to places that you were previously going to regularly. Many addicts only hang out with other addicts, and the same goes for alcoholics. If you seriously want to recover from addiction, you cannot be around people who are using drugs or alcohol. You need to develop a new circle of friends. Churches are great places to meet new friends. Make friends at AA meetings and there are recovery events where you can meet hundreds of other people who are also on the path to recovery.

There can be difficult situations within family settings where one or all members of the family are drinking alcohol or using heavy drugs. This can be a trigger for an addict in recovery. If your family members use drugs and alcohol, try to avoid attending family events completely, at least until you are out of the early stages of recovery. Skip the family gathering at Thanksgiving if you are likely to be sitting next to a family member who is getting drunk on alcohol or witnessing family members sneaking around out back to smoke illicit drugs. Just avoid the whole situation until you have at least six months of solid recovery.

## 2.4: Do Not "Do a Little" Drugs or Alcohol

Many addicts have a major relapse when they convince themselves that they can "do a little" without falling back into their addiction. Perhaps they have a day, a week, or a couple of months of clean time under their belt. They convince themselves that they have got their addiction under control, so they think it is fine to "do a little." This is dangerous thinking, and it can be fatal!

If you are an addict, you are an addict for the rest of your life. You can never do drugs or alcohol again, regardless of the amount. Complete abstinence is a simple concept to understand. You might not like the concept, but you can understand it.

Be honest with yourself that you are an addict, which means you are not able to control your consumption of drugs or alcohol. If you view this as the "hand you have been dealt," accepting complete abstinence from drugs and alcohol as the solution is simple.

The use of one drug can quickly lead to the use of another drug. Don't fool yourself into thinking you can smoke weed but not smoke meth or that you can take a dose of Valium but not a dose of opiates. One drug will lead to another, and soon you will be back to your drug of choice.

Do not engage in sneaky behavior to take your drug of choice in secret—you are lying to yourself. It is not hard to fool other people in the short term. If you engage in sneaky behavior, you will know that you are cheating, and this will undermine your self-worth. It would be more honest for you to acknowledge to yourself that you have had a small relapse. If you continue your sneaky behavior, using "a little" will lead to using more. It may take a few hours or a few days, but you will end up back where you were before, and worse still, you may try to use the same amount as you did before you got clean and overdose.

All the gains you made from the time and energy you have invested into quitting, will disappear, if you "do a little."

## 2.5: Do Not Get Into Serious Relationships

Addicts in recovery are in a fight for their life. You need to gain control of your own life before you try to include another person in your life. A romantic relationship is a major stress point for most people, and it can cause a relapse more than anything else. Avoid serious relationships when you are new to recovery because they will not help your chances of successfully recovering from addiction.

Most sexual relationships fall apart at some point, and the breakdown usually causes heartache, anger, anxiety, frustration, and stress to both parties involved. These emotions may send you running back to your drug of choice for comfort. Any kind of sexual relationship is a serious relationship, and serious relationships are dangerous for people in early recovery.

It is unrealistic for someone to succeed in recovery while having a serious relationship with another person who is using drugs or alcohol. A couple may be drinking together or shooting heroin together. If one person in the relationship wants to get clean and sober, they must leave the relationship.

Co-dependency is an excessive reliance on the other person in the relationship for your own sense of identity. These relationships are common among addicts, and they are toxic. A relationship like this can only hurt your ability to recover from addiction. Many professionals within the field of addiction believe that an addict has a co-dependent relationship with their drug of choice. All codependent relationships should be terminated.

Humans are social animals—very few humans thrive in isolation. Some can tolerate isolation better than others, but most people seek relationships. Our ability to have mutually beneficial relationships with other people is a large determinant of our personal success and happiness in life, and it is also the reason the human species has thrived on earth relative to all other animal species. For an addict in early recovery, relationships should be friendly, light, casual, positive, and playful. Definitely not sexual nor co-dependent.

Many employers are supportive of employees who are in recovery. Your relationship with your employer can be healthy and professional if honesty is a core principle within your relationship. Light, casual relationships are helpful because they don't bring stress the same way that serious relationships do. Professional relationships with therapists and drug counselors are also healthy and encouraged.

Relationships with parents and siblings can be very complicated. These relationships are also important, and the people within the relationships cannot be replaced by others. Throughout life, we go through various stages in our relationships with our families. Children are very dependent on their parents. Adolescents go through a stage of rebelling against their parents and as adults, we realize we are very similar to our parents. Most addicts have a complicated relationship with their parents and siblings. If these relationships have been stressful for you in the past, you should avoid them while you are in early recovery. I recommend you seek professional help from a counselor or therapist if you have had complicated family relationships. Get at least six months of clean time before you re-engage in complicated family relationships.

Take an honest look at your relationships with your parents, siblings, close friends, and past lovers. Write down the positives and negatives of each relationship. You will begin to discover the patterns in your relationships.

In recovery from addiction, you must take control of your own life and take responsibility for your addiction. You will be better off if you put serious relationships on hold until you have full control of yourself, and even then, you should be very careful about who you allow into your life.

# 2.6: Death, Injury and Disease

Drugs and alcohol cause significant amounts of deaths in the U.S.A. Each year, approximately two million Americans die, and approximately 5% of those deaths, or one out of every twenty deaths, are officially recorded to have been caused by drug overdose or alcohol. However, these statistics are an under representation because a pedestrian being killed by a drunk driver is recorded as a vehicle-induced death and suicide is recorded as suicide but drug addicts make up a big proportion of suicides.

Many young people are not scared of dying because they think, *Life will be over, why should I care?* They don't consider the possibility that their life may not be over and they might be left with a major injury or a debilitating condition. Many road accidents occur due to people driving drunk. If there is a car accident, people can be paralyzed or sustain head injuries that do not kill them but leave them in a compromised state for the rest of their lives. Drugs and alcohol cause many deaths, but they cause far more injuries than deaths.

Some drug-related injuries, such as poor dental health, happen as a slow onset of disease. For example, the tooth enamel of a meth addict becomes decayed from smoking their toxic drug. They get cavities, and their teeth fall out. Dentures are often required, but they can be expensive. Many addicts end up chewing on their gums for years, which can hurt, cause gum disease, and become the start of a systemic infection that affects their entire body.

A person injecting heroin with a shared needle may not die from an overdose. Instead, they may get hepatitis from the shared needle, then suffer with that disease for the rest of their life.

I had a client in his sixties who was living homeless, drinking heavily, and using meth so he could keep drinking for days at a time. One day, he had a heart attack that scared him straight for a few months. Instead of killing him, it left him weaker, more vulnerable, and unable to protect himself while living homeless on the streets.

Removing drugs and alcohol from your life doesn't just reduce your chances of death, it also reduces your risk of injury and disease while you are still alive.

Plan a "get clean date," stop using drugs and alcohol, detoxify and stay clean and sober by following the actions identified in the next chapter.

The principles identified in this chapter will help you to get through the first few days after you stop using drugs and alcohol. To get you through the first six months, follow the principles discussed in the next chapter.

# Part 3: Early Recovery - Physical Actions

To achieve success in recovery from addiction, take the <u>actions</u> listed below. These are <u>physical actions</u>. You don't have to think too much, <u>just do it.</u>

If you want to keep things simple, simply follow these actions!

These actions will increase your chances of success in recovery from addiction. If you cannot achieve all of them, do what you can. The idea is to increase your chances of success by implementing as many of these <u>actions</u> as possible.

# 3.1: Live with Sober People

After detox, do not return to the environment you were living in while you were using—whether that was the streets, your car, your parents' house, a place you shared with "friends," your own apartment, or any other place where you used drugs or alcohol regularly.

I highly recommend that you live with other people who are also recovering from addiction. A well-run sober home is a good choice—the camaraderie and peer-to-peer support you will receive are valuable. There will be other people living there with more clean time than you. They can relate to what you are going through and they can give you an example to follow.

Living with sober people is my first recommendation for early recovery because I believe it is the most important action you can take to improve your chances of success in staying off drugs and alcohol permanently!

A sober living environment (SLE) is a home where you must agree to abide by the structures that have been put in place in order to assist your recovery from addiction. The most notable of these is zero tolerance of illicit drugs and alcohol. Most SLE's will not admit you without your agreement to leave the sober home within one hour, if you relapse. This helps the other people who are living in the sober home to maintain their sobriety and not be triggered back into addiction by somebody else's relapse.

You should think of your sober home as <u>your home</u> and the people who live there as <u>your family</u> for the duration of the time you live there. However, the people that run the sober home are not your parents, and they are not going to beg you follow the rules. If you don't fit into the structure, you will be given a warning or two before being asked to leave so that the sober home can function as it is intended to function, which is a sober home for people who are serious about overcoming their addictions.

Don't expect the people who run the sober home to do the hard work for you. You are responsible for your own recovery. The sober home is there to provide you with a good environment to help you do the work you need to do in order to maintain your sobriety and get your life back on track.

You should live in a sober home for at least six months, if you find yourself improving, stay there longer. Those who have gotten the most out of our sober living home have lived here for several years. Becoming part of the management team that is running the sober home is an excellent way to learn about the difficulties other addicts face on their journeys to recovery. Most sober living homes have many opportunities for clients to be of service, and you will get more out of your time living in a sober home if you look for ways to be of service to the sober home.

## 3.2: Go to Recovery Meetings

I highly recommend that you go to recovery meetings as a vital part of your recovery program. These meetings are particularly helpful in early recovery, as well as after many years of sobriety. It is reassuring to see other people dealing with the same struggles you are dealing with because it makes you realize that you are not alone.

Some addicts in early recovery commit to attend ninety meetings, in ninety days. This is an excellent start. You are likely to make new friends at these meetings, so you can begin to replace your old "circle of addicts" with a "circle of friends" who can offer you support to stay clean and sober.

After you have been clean and sober for several months, you might not feel the need to go to recovery meetings as much as you did in early recovery. Do not stop going to meetings altogether because this is a common precursor to a relapse. I have heard many people share about how their meeting attendance declined prior to their relapse.

I found Alcoholics Anonymous (AA) meetings to be my favorite recovery meeting mostly because there are several in my neighborhood and there are many people there who are my age and whom I considered to be my peers. Narcotics Anonymous (NA) meetings were also helpful to me. I also attended other recovery meetings like Smart Recovery, Buddha Recovery, and Al-Anon (a support group for people who love an addict), as well as recovery events such as Recovery Happens, which is a two-day, convention-style event attended by thousands of people in recovery.

Make sure you participate in recovery meetings when you attend them. When you are new, let other people start the meeting so that you can get comfortable with how the meeting is conducted, then contribute to the meeting with your input. People who are new to recovery can add fresh insight that helps the "old goats" keep up their efforts in recovery. Everyone is there to help each other and everybody's input matters, so make sure you participate. You can share your thoughts with the group and use the opportunity to "shine the light of honesty" onto your struggles, which is likely to make your struggles more tolerable.

Many addicts will "isolate and medicate." One of the characteristics of being an addict is using drugs and alcohol while alone. You should not isolate when you are in early recovery. It is not wise to have prolonged isolation from other people. Once you are done with your initial detox period, get out and about. Recovery meetings are a great way to get out and meet people.

A recovery meeting is a relatively safe place for you to interact with others, although you should be aware in advance that there are times when a person will attend a recovery meeting while loaded. Depending on the group, the meeting secretary may ask that person to leave, but they may not if they believe the loaded person is trying to move in the right direction. Allow the meeting secretary to make this decision. In everyday society, you have to maintain your self-control while in the company of other people who are loaded, so experiencing this at a sobriety meeting is a safe place to gain some practice.

**Direction:** Make a list of the recovery meetings you will attend.

_____

_____

_____

_____

_____

_____

_____

_____

_____

_____

_____

_____

_____

_____

# 3.3: Talk - Shine a Light on the Darkness

While it may be difficult, talking honestly to other people about your deep thoughts and feelings can be extremely healthy and beneficial for you. From my own experience, I have found that talking to people about difficult topics or emotions takes power away from the topic or emotion and leaves me feeling better and mentally stronger. Bottling up difficult issues and never talking about them has the opposite effect, giving the issues more power over you.

This does not mean that I recommend airing your dirty laundry in public. You should not use Facebook or other social media platforms to tell the world about your problems. You should not talk to most of your friends about your deeper problems either because they may not know what to say, they may give bad advice or they may gossip with others about what you've told them and break your trust, which will hurt you further.

Talking about your feelings and actions is a good reason to attend and participate in recovery meetings because you can discuss your problems with peers who have faced similar issues. Everyone attending the meeting agrees to keep the meeting confidential which has always been my experience.

Some people isolate in a crowd. They blend into the background or sit alone in a corner and wallow in their depression or loneliness. Do not let this be you. Get involved in recovery meetings, participate, exchange ideas, and interact with other people.

It can be helpful to identify a few people in your life whom you respect and trust to have an open, honest relationship. Politely ask them if it would be okay for you to have a talk with them about your problems and your efforts to overcome your problems.

Some of the best people to talk to about your feelings and actions are professional counselors and therapists who are trained to be good listeners and have experience guiding many other people who have faced similar problems. Don't delay making the call to these types of professionals! Many of us don't have people in our lives we can talk to about our most personal problems. Men tend to be stoic and bottle up their feelings. A strategy of "tough out bad times" is not a good strategy in our modern world. Make an appointment with a professional so that you can talk out your problems.

## 3.4: Get a Sponsor

Recovery meetings are the best place to find a sponsor. A sponsor is a mentor who will support you on your journey of recovery. Your sponsor should have more experience and knowledge about recovery from addiction than you, and they should be solid in their own recovery. You should be able to call them any time you are having cravings to use drugs or alcohol.

You should call your sponsor daily during your early recovery, even if only to check in and have a friendly chat. This can be very helpful, as they can encourage you to stay on track. You should like and respect your sponsor, and they must have time for you when you need them. Some sponsors are popular and may be sponsoring multiple people. This means that they are very busy and may have less time for you than you need.

Try not to get frustrated with your sponsor. People who are willing to mentor you do so because they are good people who want to help you. However, it can be a good idea to have more than one sponsor or at least a second person in mind as a back-up plan. If the relationship is not working out with your first sponsor, you can easily transfer to a different sponsor instead of being left with no one. Keep in mind that one sponsor may be good at a certain aspect of recovery but not others. The idea is that you always have sponsors in your corner to help you battle the temptations to use drugs and alcohol.

Once you have more than one year of sobriety and you feel like your recovery is strong, you should make yourself available to sponsor other people who are new to recovery. This can strengthen your own recovery, and it gives back to the community of people who have helped you.

**Direction:** Please write down the names of people who are a potential sponsor for you.

_____

_____

_____

_____

_____

_____

_____

_____

_____

_____

_____

_____

_____

_____

_____

_____

_____

_____

_____

# 3.5: Get a Job - It Provides Structure

During your recovery, it is very important that you get a paid job. I recommend that you start with an entry-level job or a minimum wage job because they are lower stress and easier to get and you can start working immediately. Also, entry level jobs have more opportunities for positive progression and progress is fundamental for feeling good about yourself.

A paid job provides you with structure and routine. You can build relationships with your co-workers and develop friendships that are not centered around drugs and alcohol. You might also end up with some disposable income since you are no longer wasting your money on drugs and alcohol. For the last couple of decades, California has had more than enough jobs available for anyone seriously looking for a job.

Doing college classes or volunteer work is not a substitute for a paid job, and you should not be working for a relative that is giving you "protected employment." You need regular work hours and a defined set of tasks that you are expected to perform for an organization that is not treating you any differently from how it treats all of its other employees. The structure and daily routine of a job that forces you to interact with work colleagues is particularly helpful for people in recovery.

I recommend that you inform your employer that you are recovering from addiction. Informing your employer, especially during an initial interview, immediately establishes a honest relationship. This will serve you well over time. Hiding this information from your employer is a lie by omission and has the opposite effect.

You should not be looking for your dream job—an entry-level or minimum wage job is a better option. If you start in an entry-level position, you are more likely to have opportunities for growth. Starting from the bottom and showing you have a strong work ethic and can hold down your position reliably will make your employer more likely to consider you for a promotion or help you to leverage a better job at the different company later.

When you start in an entry-level position, there is no pressure on you to make a long-term commitment to your employer. If you work the job for a few months and don't like it, find another job and give that a try. Use this period to try out different working environments. If you like the idea of working outside, you could apply for positions in tree cutting, construction, or delivery driving. Perhaps you'd prefer to work in an office doing computer work, accounting, or office administration.

Trade work is an excellent choice for a lot of recovering addicts. Trade jobs for plumbers, electricians, carpenters, landscapers, roofers and painters are always open for new applicants. The work is usually physically demanding, but the independence is attractive. These jobs pay well, particularly as your skills increase. Trade jobs give you the possibility to build you own business and have a profitable career. If you achieve long-term sobriety, I encourage you to consider starting your own business but in early recovery, the structure of a paid job is your primary goal.

Some jobs are isolating by the nature of the work. For example, computer programming can cause the programmer to have little interaction with other people because they have their "head in a computer" all day long. The same goes for working the "graveyard" shift, which isolates you because it puts you on a very different schedule from most other people. If your job is isolating you from society, you may need to find a new job as part of your plan for recovery from addiction.

If you have been a long-term addict and have worked in one particular industry during that time, clearly this industry has not served you well, even though you may know the industry well and you may be able to find work easily within it. Don't go back to the same job and the same people, and think that you are going to get a different result. Try something new.

Your goal should be to get any job to start with and over time work towards better jobs that are a better fit for you—with each job being better than the last. This approach allows you to start working quickly and build a plan for your long-term goals over time. You get structure into your life quickly and you can start saving some money for your future.

**Direction:** Please write down the jobs which interest you?

_____

_____

_____

_____

_____

_____

_____

_____

_____

_____

_____

_____

_____

_____

_____

_____

_____

_____

_____

# 3.6: Get Healthy

Most addicts in early recovery need to improve their health, which I have broken down into:

3.6.1:   Breath
3.6.2:   Drink
3.6.3:   Eat
3.6.4:   Sleep
3.6.5:   Hygiene
3.6.6:   Appearance
3.6.7:   Exercise

---

### 3.6.1: Breath:

Very few people are breathing with good technique and almost everyone can improve. If we don't breath, we will die in less than 5 minutes. After your heart beating, breathing is the most critical body function and most of us do not breath with optimal technique.

Ideally you should breath in through your nose and fill your lungs from the bottom of your stomach up to the top of your chest, then open your mouth and exhale with a relaxed open throat. Pause and repeat.

The importance of proper breathing is under appreciated because we get used to our breathing habits and it is hard to notice our poor technique. This is why you should attended breathing workshops. These sessions are similar to yoga or meditation sessions but the focus is on breathing and most classes are structured to encourage the student to hyperventilate, maximizing the oxygen levels in your blood and creating a peak experience during the class. This peak can bring great clarity of mind. There is normally a calm down period where the student decreases their breathing and will often fall asleep or go into a dream like state. I encourage you to do a breath work class once a month.

I know that this point is going to be unpopular with most readers because the vast majority of people recovering from addiction either smoke cigarettes or use a vape. This likely includes you. Don't fool yourself, smoking is breathing in chemicals which are bad for your health. You should eliminate this harmful addiction from your life.

If it is too much for you to stop smoking while quitting drugs and alcohol, come up with a plan to quit smoking as a next step. If you can quit drugs and alcohol, you can quit cigarettes. I have a colleague who smoked cigarettes and shot heroin for twenty years, then quit heroin with the help of Suboxone and switched the cigarettes for a vape with a nicotine fluid. Then, he titrated down the nicotine content in the fluid to zero over a period of one year and stopped vaping completely. Today, he has many years clean and sober and many months of no smoking. You can do this to or come up with your own plan to quit smoking.

Breathing clean air into big lungs will improve your health.

## 3.6.2: Drink:

If you don't drink fluids you will die in approximately 5 days. The best hydration is clean water. I like refrigerated, carbonated water, in a can, with zero calories. To me this feels and tastes great. I also like bottled water, mineral water and water from a clean stream.

Do not drink sugary sodas, fruit juices or fancy coffee drinks which are mostly sugar. You are taking in calories that have very little nutritional value. Sugary drinks confuse the decision to hydrate with the rewards from sugar intake. Don't do this. Stop before you purchase a 12-pack of soda or a Super Sized drink at a fast food outlet. These drinks are empty calories that make you fat.

Your urine should be a pale yellow color. Dark yellow means that you are de-hydrated and need to drink more clean water. De-hydration is common as many people do not drink enough clean water. Colorless urine means that you are over hydrated and that you should drink less.

## 3.6.3: Eat:

I recommend that you remove all ultra processed foods and most simple carbohydrates from your diet. Processed foods normally come in a box or plastic container. This includes popular items such as TV dinners, processed meats, cereal, muffins, bread and so on. Eat natural foods, food made by nature before they are processed by humans. These foods are healthier for you.

Removing most simple carbohydrates from your diet means removing sugar, candy, soda, ice cream, pasta, rice, bread, grains, potatoes, biscuits, cookies and so on. These simple carbohydrates are metabolized into glucose, which are then quickly absorbed into your bloodstream, combined with insulin and stored as fat, leaving you feeling hungry again a few hours after you have eaten and more prone to inflammation through-out your body. The spike in your blood sugar results in your body producing excessive insulin to control the sugar and the glucose plus insulin is stored as fat. This sets up a cycle in your body of highs and lows that affect your mood.

Your brain is mostly made up of fat. Eating a high-fat diet may support brain function. Many people in early recovery from addiction have independently decided to follow the Keto diet (a high-fat, low-carb diet that includes leafy green vegetables). This is a good diet for the first 6-24 months of recovery as it may help your brain to settle into a new normal. Later, you may want to transition to a greater percentage of vegetables (70%) with some natural fats(20%) and proteins (10%). A diet with a high percentage of vegetables and a very diverse group of vegetables, for example more than 30 different vegetables in one week, may help you to become slimmer. A lightly heated stir fry consisting of diverse organic vegetables cooked in virgin olive oil with a small amount of turmeric and curry spice is an example of a healthy meal. .

I recommend that you prepare your meals at home so that you can control the ingredients and develop your personalized diet. There is not one diet for all people. People respond differently to food. You should experiment to find the diet that fits you best. It may change as you age. Most nutrition experts agree that recently harvested foods are healthier for you than foods that have been dead a long time.

A diverse gut bacteria is good for your physical and mental health. Probiotics such as yogurt (sugar free and full fat), kefir and fermented vegetables (for example sauerkraut) help to create a diverse bacteria colony in your gut. Antibiotics will kill off bacteria in your gut and these should only be taken under medical supervision. Creating a happy gut and a digestive system that is functioning well should be your goal with food.

It is important to stop snacking because snacking causes an eating pattern of constant "grazing." Often, the food being snacked on is made up of simple carbohydrates with loads of preservatives and sugar. Snack foods are often found in a plastic wrapper with misleading marketing messages such as "health bar". If a food has been put through a mechanical process, crushed, pressurized, heated, and mixed with additives to keep it stable so that it has a longer shelf life, it is not a health food.

Consider doing intermittent fasting, which is basically when you eat only two meals a day. Eat your first meal at 10 a.m. and your last meal at 4 p.m. with no snacking in between. This meal plan provides a fasting period of eighteen hours from 4 p.m. until 10 a.m. the next day. Having this fasting period each day is very healthy because it takes approximately sixteen hours for your liver to distribute all of its glucose into your bloodstream, which then gives you two hours to burn fat each day. Ideally, your body will start burning fat for fuel rather than glucose. When this happens, your body can draw down on the energy stored in your fat cells. You may lose some excess body fat, enjoy longer periods without feeling hungry, and improve your mood.

If eating two meals a day is easy for you, try eating only one meal a day. This is called the one meal a day (OMAD) diet. Most people struggle to do this consistently, so start slowly and see if you can work your way toward eating less meals each day with no snacks in between meals.

Also, consider doing longer fasts for 7-21 days. You should have medical supervision or at least someone who can check on you throughout the day. Most people who have tried fasting for longer periods have found it to be very beneficial. The main benefits of long-term fasting is the elimination of toxins and excretion of waste from the cells of your body. Long-term fasting also elevates mood, reduces depression and resets the expression of genes produced by multiple organs.

After three days of fasting, most people no longer feel any hunger because their bodies have converted to burning body fat as fuel. It is a good idea to avoid expending unnecessary energy during longer fasting periods. Longer fasting periods should be dedicated to fasting, with very little other activities taking place. Keep your activities light. This helps the digestive system to remain dormant. When the fasting period ends, there should be a slow, measured reintroduction to food, not a sudden binge. This allows the digestive system to start working again.

Heavy exercise or hard physical labor will make you hungry and you are much more likely to eat sugar and carbohydrates when you become very hungry. Men who work hard physical labor jobs for ten years or more, tend to get heavier as they age because they are burning a large amount of calories, they have to eat large amounts of food. Slim people tend to eat much less food and burn much less calories. Slim people tend to live longer too.

The digestive tract ends at your anus and it is important to have regular movement within your digestive tract. Constipation increase the amount of toxins your organs have to handle. It is desirable to eliminate daily within a hour of waking up. Meal planning should include consideration of daily elimination. Magnesium tablets will cause a bowel movement and lower your blood pressure. A monthly purge of your digestive system has many health benefits. It can be achieved by drinking castor oil, magnesium tablets, other laxatives and colonic enemas.

Your digestive tract is a major part of your over-all health and it should be given attention from it's beginning, your mouth and teeth, to it's middle section which is your stomach, intestines and energy absorption organs, to it's end, which is your colon and anus. Take a holistic approach. If your digestive system is working well, your ability to overcome your addiction is increased.

## 3.6.4: Sleep:

Sleep and adequate rest are important for people who are overcoming addiction, but that does not mean lying around all day doing nothing! Eight hours of sleep is plenty, but if you feel like you need more, go ahead, as long as you are awake, properly dressed, and doing something productive during the day.

Going to bed a few hours after the sun has gone down is recommended. If you are in recovery, it is important to match your daily routine with the daylight hours. Be sure to set your daily sleep cycle in coordination with the darkest hours. Avoid doing night work, particularly the graveyard shift from midnight to 6am. Working those hours will reduce your time in the daylight, which is bad for your mental health. There are work opportunities at night which often pay more in order to incentivize people to do them but if you are an addict in recovery from addiction, these work opportunities are not good for you. You should synchronize your lifestyle with the sun.

Most sleep experts recommend keeping a consistent sleep schedule, which means going to bed at the same time each night. Good sleep is vital to good health. Putting effort into getting good sleep is worth your time and making your bed in the morning is part of a good sleep routine. You should also be settling down before bed, preparing your sleeping area to be comfortable, turning off mental stimulants such as electronic devices, screens and bright lights, and not consuming stimulants, such as caffeine, for several hours before bedtime.

**3.6.5: Hygiene:**

Be sure to take care of your personal hygiene as a conscious decision and a practiced physical action. Taking a shower at least three times a week, washing your hair with shampoo, and brushing your teeth are important parts of your daily routine that leave you feeling good and smelling better.

Oral hygiene is important. Give your mouth and teeth some tender loving care with dental floss and toothpaste. Mercury amalgam fillings are an old technology that should be replaced with new "white fillings" if possible. There are people who believe that the mercury in these old fillings leaks into your body tissue and can cause multiple complications to your health. It is unclear if this is true but if the opportunities arises to replace old mercury fillings, it should be taken. Many people in recovery have neglected their dental hygiene, so their teeth are in poor condition. If this is the case for you, consider setting a goal of getting dental work done if you can stay off drugs and alcohol for a period of time. Reward yourself and start the process of improving your teeth. Not only will you look better, but you will be able to eat better too.

Being clean takes little effort and makes you feel good about yourself. It is hard to develop a positive self-image if you are dirty or smell bad. During addiction, basic personal hygiene is often neglected. While running my sober home, I have told multiple clients that they must take a shower because other clients have complained to the management team about their bad odor.

If you are going to be successful in recovering from addiction, you must have good personal hygiene practices. This is a physical action. Get into your new, clean and sober hygiene routines as conscious physical actions that you take every day.

**3.6.6: Appearance:**

I highly recommend that you give yourself a makeover. Clean yourself up, change your hairstyle, and dress well. This does not need to cost much. It is mostly that you need to make a conscious decision to change your outward appearance.

Many professional workers wear specific uniforms which make them easily identifiable: firefighters, police officers, doctors, nurses, tradesmen, business-people, etc. Most drug addicts and alcoholics wear a "uniform" too. The most common item of clothing worn by drug addicts is a black hoodie, worn with a baseball cap and the hoodie up. If you are going to change to a new lifestyle, you should strongly consider changing your clothes to reflect your new mindset. If you have not used drugs or alcohol for several days but you are still wearing the same clothes you wore while you were using, your chances of relapse are very high because you are in the same place that you were when you were using drugs.

The way you walk and carry yourself should also change. Have you heard the expression "drunken stagger." There is also a "heroin nod out," a "speed freak jitter" and a "pimp limp?" Try to be self-aware about how you carry yourself and make sure you practice good body posture. Stand up straight, put a smile on your face, raise your chin up so that you are not constantly looking down at the ground, and speak in a clear voice. This improves your appearance and it benefits you.

Thrift stores offer excellent clothes at a low cost, so they are a good place to start shopping for new clothes. A haircut, a shave, and a shower do not cost much. Be honest with yourself, your previous lifestyle choices did not work well for you, right? So don't hang onto them. Change them. It is your physical actions to change and carry yourself with dignity which is required to assist your recovery from addiction.

## 3.6.7: Exercise:

Gentle exercise is good for everyone, but it can be especially helpful to addicts in recovery. Walking is the best option for gentle exercise. It is free and easy to do. One of the best times for a gentle walk is before breakfast. This also allows you to prolong your fasting period. You don't need to hike up the side of a mountain, just take a walk around your neighborhood. Another good time to walk is in the evening after your last meal of the day. Walking throughout the day is also a good idea. Some other gentle exercise options are swimming, yoga, stretching and breathing exercises.

I do not recommend any intensive exercise until you reach at least six months of solid recovery because the stress on your body and the endorphins released may trigger you to relapse. Hard-core exercise includes heavy weight training. I have seen a surprising number of drug addicts who train hard and their weight training becomes a substitute addiction. Because most drug addicts are familiar with injections and pills, taking steroids to improve their gym performance is an easy step for most drug addict to take. Many addicts are willing to admit their addiction to illicit drugs, but they will lie about their steroid use. If you are an addict in recovery and you are using steroids, you have simply swapped one addiction for another. Get off steroids and stop the heavy weight training.

Your exercise should not include any high-adrenaline activities like parachuting, BASE jumping, or wing-suit flying. In general, high-adrenaline activities do not help your recovery. You will do better with calm activities and light exercises like walking, swimming, or doing press-ups, sit-ups, and squats.

## 3.7: Polite Manners - For Your Benefit

Learning how to be polite is important for your benefit, not for the benefit of the other person to whom you are being polite. When other people perceive you as polite, they treat you better. Practice being polite as a physical action. Hold doors open and speak kind words as physical actions to train your behavior.

There are many ways to be polite, saying "please" and "thank you" is a great place to start. Some people claim that "please" and "thank you" are the three most important words in the world. In my opinion, the most important word to every person is their name. Remembering a person's name and saying that name politely when you talk to them is a powerful method of being polite. Use the words "sir" or "madam" to address a man or woman whose name you do not know. Holding doors open for others, allowing other people into traffic while driving, and not rushing ahead of other people are all good ways to be polite.

These are not situations of allowing other people to take advantage of you. They are opportunities for you to remind yourself that you are a love-abled person who deserves to be respected by other people. Being polite and considerate to other people is something you train yourself to do for your benefit! Don't expect immediate gratification every time you are polite. You have to be polite out of habit, then your reward will come slowly over time.

Another important piece of being polite is knowing when to say "I apologize" to avoid a needless confrontation. Be sure to state specifically what you are apologizing for and be sincere in your intention and tone of voice. When you apologize to someone, do not mumble or act timid. Instead, hold your head up high, stand up straight, and speak in a clear voice. Other people will respect you for it, and more importantly, you will hold yourself in a higher regard for having done it. Apologizing is much better than getting into a fight about who was "right." You are not apologizing for the benefit of the other person but for your benefit, since you avoid unnecessary stress and can move on with your day more quickly and with more dignity.

It is not hard to train yourself to be polite and once you are in the habit of being polite, it will become automatic. Then, "magically," other people will treat you better.

## 3.8: Help Others and Be of Service

Helping others and contributing positively to your community will bring a huge improvement to your life. Genuine giving creates happiness.

Much of our suffering is a by-product of our feelings of separation and lack of connection to our communities. If you are feeling depressed, help other people. You are more likely to feel happy. If you reach out to people who are less fortunate than yourself, you will find it easier to count your blessings. Keep company with someone who is sick or bedridden. Reach out to someone who is ignored by most of society. Walk around your local neighborhood and look for elderly, homeless, disabled, or poor people and treat them with kindness. It will benefit them and it will help you to feel better about your own circumstances.

If you consistently provide services to other people and you are consistently helpful to your community, you will be liked by other people. This will help you to feel genuinely good about yourself, which in turn will help you stay on track with your recovery from addiction.

Selflessly helping others will also prevent your ego from getting too big. Having a big ego can lead you to feel overconfident that you have beat your addiction, and this can lead to a relapse. Stay humble by being of service to your community and to the people who are less fortunate than you.

One of the easiest ways for you to be of service is to help at the sober home where you live or the AA, NA, or other recovery meetings that you attend. Volunteer for a service position, such as coffee service or chair set up, or volunteer to become part of the management team of your sober living home.

**Direction:** Please write down how you will help others and be of service to your community.

_____

_____

_____

_____

_____

_____

_____

_____

_____

_____

_____

_____

_____

_____

_____

_____

_____

_____

# 3.9: Develop Your Own Program of Recovery

I am a big supporter of all the Alcoholics Anonymous programs (AA, NA and Al-Anon). The basic building blocks of AA are their recovery meetings, the twelve-step program, and service to the recovery community. There are many other recovery programs that are also valuable, including Intensive Out-Patient (IOP) programs, SMART Recovery, Buddha Recovery, Conscious Recovery, Spiritual Recovery, and Religious Recovery.

I encourage you to try as many of these programs as you can to see which ones work best for you. Recovery programs are not a case of "one size fits all," so you must put effort into finding what works best for you.

Learn from each of these programs and begin to develop your own program of recovery. Make it suitable for your lifestyle. Clearly define your program of recovery. Write it down and review it with your sponsor so that you can be confident you're on the right track. If you develop your own program, really work at it, and take responsibility for it, you are more likely to succeed at your recovery from addiction.

You must develop a program of recovery that is a good fit for you, so that you can easily maintain your program of recovery and stay off drugs and alcohol permanently.

In summary, this chapter focused on physical actions that you can take to improve your chances of success in your recovery from addiction. The following chapter will focus on taking control of your mind for your long term success in recovery from addiction.

**Direction:** Please write down your Program of Recovery. What does it look like?

_____

_____

_____

_____

_____

_____

_____

_____

_____

_____

_____

_____

_____

_____

_____

_____

_____

_____

_____

_____

_____

# Part 4: Long Term Recovery - Control Your Mind

The key to long-term sobriety is to control of your mind!

Taking control of your own mind is also the key to a good life in general, not just long-term sobriety. Not only drug addicts and alcoholics have a problem with self-control, many personality types have this struggle. Anyone who wants to have a fulfilling life must control of their own mind.

The principles listed below will help you to take control of your mind. I encourage you to practice these principles every day. Repetition is key to creating a new normal for yourself.

Never compare yourself to others. Instead, compare yourself to the person you were yesterday or last month. Are you improving?

Keep practicing the principles identified below. You will improve. It may take months or years to notice your improvements, but you will notice them. They will be real improvements and other people will notice them too.

## 4.1: Love Is Your Answer

"LOVE" is the answer to all your questions! I want to emphasize this as much as possible, the answer to all your questions is LOVE!

Here is one mantra that will assist you more than any other:

**LOVE ALL PEOPLE
including the stupid things
they do and say!**

Look for the positive qualities in other people and try to disregard their negative qualities. Even love the people who have hurt you! This is tough, but it is important that you try because you need to love everyone around you in order to love yourself fully. Keep reinforcing this attitude to yourself so that, over time, you can feel love toward all people, including yourself.

When you are focused on feeling love for everyone and everything, you reinforce positive emotions in your mind. You are the one feeling the positive emotions and you are the one who benefits from them. This is why you should try your best to feel love toward all people because you will benefit from those feelings of love.

Human experience happens from the inside, all your emotions (love, joy, fear and anger) are felt inside your mind. The seat of your experience is inside your mind and you must take control of your mind.

Your positive emotions can be felt by those you interact with and can influence their mood positively. People who feel your positive energy may return this energy to you, creating a positive feedback loop.

Keep your expectations of yourself and others low. When high expectations art not met, you will feel frustration and anger. Low expectations will help you feel love for others and yourself. I recommend that you care for yourself as you would care for someone you love. Don't be hard on yourself. Love yourself in a humble way, as best you can.

The person who needs your love the most is you! You must love yourself before it is reasonable for you to expect some-one else to love you. Feel within yourself that you are deeply loved and cared for by yourself. Tell yourself that you have nothing to be afraid of.

Bring this mindset of love to how you look at your mistakes. Take them seriously and learn from them. Make a commitment to not repeat your mistakes, then put them behind you and move forward with love in your heart. Do not be too hard on yourself. It is unnecessary and does not help you.

On your journey of recovery, you will have many questions like "How do I talk to my family about my actions while I was in addiction?" or "How do I interact with my ex-lover whom I treated badly?" The answer to all these questions is "with love."

Most people who have struggled with addiction have made many stupid mistakes. A lot of addicts will have lied, cheated, stolen from relatives and promised the world but delivered dirt. If you feel it is hard to love yourself, start by forgiving yourself.

Be sure not to blame your bad actions on other people or circumstances because you do not want a victim mentality. Take responsibility for your actions and own your actions but don't be a prisoner to your past. Ask yourself for forgiveness, then move forward with a commitment to never repeat the actions that you know to be a mistake.

Think about the positive qualities you see in yourself. Write them down and start building your self-love by acknowledging your most positive strengths. In my opinion, you will get further, faster by playing to your strengths, rather than focusing on your weaknesses. However, that does not mean you should sweep your negative traits under the carpet. If you want to build a positive self-image, spend 90% of your time focusing on building your strengths and the other 10% of your effort on improving your weaknesses.

Include yourself in your attitude of love toward all people. Start by loving yourself for your strengths and love all people as best you can.

## 4.2: Honesty Is Essential

Being honest with yourself and others is a big step on the way to taking control of your mind. Like an onion, there are layers to honesty. Peeling back one layer leads to another layer that could not be accessed before.

Honesty _must_ become the central pillar on which you build yourself. First, learn to be honest with yourself. Many addicts suffer from delusions of grandeur, thinking they are sexy, smart, or successful with no evidence to support their thoughts. Many addicts lie to themselves for years about the life they lead. It is easy for them to lie to other people because they have become very good at lying to themselves. To break this cycle, an addict should be honest with themself and everyone else.

Being honest about the number of drugs you were (or are) using or the amount of alcohol you were (or are) consuming is a good starting point. Take an honest look at your lifestyle. Look at your financial situation and your ability to earn an income to support yourself. Whether you like it or not, making money is an important part of life. Everyone needs to be honest with themselves about their ability to make money.

After yourself, the next group of people to be honest with is your loved ones. Start with the people that you care about most and have honest conversations with them about your addiction and your efforts at recovery from addiction.

I recommend that you inform your employer that you are recovering from addiction. An employer-employee relationship is an important relationship and it should be based on honesty, and this honesty must include not withholding important information. Some employers have a program to help employees with recovery from addiction. If you have a job that can impact the safety of other people, such as being a driver or airline pilot, and you are abusing alcohol or drugs, informing your employer is the responsible action to take even if you lose your job. Innocent people can get killed because of your chemical dependency. You must inform your employer and get help for yourself.

Living an honest life is an essential foundation for your recovery from addiction. I encourage you to take control of your mind and make a conscious decision to live an honest life.

## 4.3: Learn to Say "No"

In order to overcome addiction, you have to say "NO!" to drugs and alcohol. Use this as an opportunity to practice saying "no" to people and ideas too.

"No" is a small, two letter word with a big meaning. Many people are not good at saying "no" mostly because they want to be liked. People say "yes" because they want to conform and because they know that everyone asking them a question wants to hear a "yes" answer. People also say "yes" because they want to go with the flow or run with the herd. Being agreeable has its place but this must be balanced with what is in your best interest.

A child may cry when they do not get what they want, but at some point, the child needs to grow up. There has to be a realization by the child that it cannot have everything they want. The concept of "no" has to be learned. Otherwise, the result is a child in an adult's body.

It is good practice for an addict to say "no" to the requests of others if those requests are too great or inconvenient for some reason. Simple, polite words can be used. Saying "no, I am not available now" is far better than saying "yes" and not following through.

Saying "no" generally leaves more power with the person saying "no." Saying "yes" generally means you have a desire to be liked.

The next time someone sings out your name in a sweet tone of voice, be prepared to hear that person ask you for something. While they are making their request, prepare yourself to give them a polite "no, not today, thank you." I guarantee you that no one will ever sing out your name, then offer to do something for your benefit. It will always be that they are going to ask you for something. Just say, "No, not today, thank you." Sometimes you may choose to soften your "no" with words that are designed to make the other person feel good. For example you may say "I would love to help you but I have other commitments" or "thank you for thinking about me, unfortunately I am un-available". Using soft words is a secondary consideration. The primary point is to learn the skill of saying "no" when you are asked to do something that is not in your best interests.

I am not recommending that you become a grumpy, disagreeable person or that you never help other people. Helping others is good for you, but you choose the time, place, and type of help. You take control into your hands. Learn to say "no" to the requests of others, then help people at a time and in a manner that you choose.

I recommend that you stop trying to be liked by everyone. You put yourself at a disadvantage if you want other people to "like you." Wanting to be liked by everyone is an impossible goal. It is never going to happen, and it puts you at a disadvantage where you are constantly trying to please other people or seek their approval. The responsibility is on you to outgrow the need to be liked by everyone.

Malevolent people exist. Some family members, friends, and strangers wish evil on you. Their malevolence is not a result of something you have done, or not done, it is a result of their shortcomings in life. Learning to say "no" to other people, helps to protect you from malevolent people.

Passive-aggressive people are not as destructive as malevolent people, but they can cause emotional and psychological pain too. As you improve your ability to say "no," your ability to identify passive-aggressive people in your life will increase. I recommend that you say "no" to them as soon as possible.

To control your mind, you must make a conscious decision to say "no" to people and ideas that are not in your best interests.

# 4.4: Voices and Personas

Most people have several voices or "personas" that play out in our minds throughout the day. For example, you may have a victim persona that starts up whenever something goes wrong. The voice may say, "Nothing ever goes right for me," "I am always losing out," or "Why can't I win?" All of us have things go wrong every day, so a person who has this voice in their mind will be influenced by it multiple times, every day.

Inner voice chatter is usually negative and self-deprecating, and it is often what drives people to use drugs and alcohol. You can lower the volume of your inner voices by asking yourself, "Who's voice is this?" and "Is this voice saying anything helpful?" You will experience more mental clarity if you can learn to quiet your inner voices.

There could be voices of anger, self-righteousness, vulnerability, pride, a desire to be loved, and many more. You must learn to take control of your relationship with these voices to gain better control of your mind.

You can start the process by identifying your voices, then lowering the "volume" of the voices that are toxic to you, especially the voice that tells you it is "okay" to use drugs and alcohol or practice your addictive behavior. Replace your negative voices by focusing on the voices that are healthy for you, such as your voices of love or your voice of helpfulness that you have been developing throughout your recovery.

This is how you take control of your center of consciousness and your life. This will give you a better handle on how other people perceive you and the content of your character. By taking control of your internal voices, personas, or identities in your mind, you can move your center of consciousness in a positive direction that will leave you feeling more content with yourself and your life.

Most people have multiple identities. It is probably that you have heard of the "Jekyll and Hyde" persona that is often present in a bad-tempered alcoholic. A person may be a lover or a fighter, a hard worker or a slacker, a brother or sister, a beast or a bitch. Many of these identities will not be peaceful in nature. Human history shows many examples of violent, extremist, and self-centered identities.

The "chatter" from all these personas is confusing. Reducing the number of personas, especially the negative personas, is helpful to you. What personas do you have? Which personas do you like the most?

Below, write down the name of the person you think of when you call to mind the specific persona listed. Who is this person? Can you visualize them? Can you name them? What do you like or dislike about this person? Try to use this information to your advantage.

Angry persona: _____

_____

Drug-addict persona: _____

_____

Alcoholic persona: _____

_____

Respectful persona: _____

_____

Peaceful persona: _____

_____

Happy persona: _____

_____

Popular psychology claims that you are the sum of the five people that you spend the most time with. Perhaps it is more correct that you are the sum of the five persona's which dominate your mind.

Sometimes a persona can be so strong that it is a major part of your identity. Many addicts have created an identity around drugs and alcohol. This identity needs to disappear completely if you are going to recover from addiction. You must shift your focus to your positive personas to facilitate the disappearance of the negative personas.

If your center of consciousness is focused on loving and helping other people, you are likely to feel more loved and fulfilled in your own life. Focus on your happy personas and you are more likely to become happy yourself.

Think of people who you admire. What do you picture? What principles do you believe they live by?

I recommend that you imagine the best version of yourself that you can, then manifest an interesting persona around this positive self-image. Who you want to become is more important than who you have been in the past. Make sure you have fun creating this persona. The world needs you with all your unique individuality, especially when you are at your best.

**Direction:** Write down your best persona. Picture yourself. Describe your look and feel. Who are you? What actions do you perform? What are your strong points?

_____

_____

_____

_____

_____

_____

_____

_____

_____

_____

_____

_____

_____

_____

_____

_____

_____

_____

# 4.5: Improve Your Spiritual Health

Spirituality is seeking a meaningful connection with something bigger than yourself.

Improving your spiritual health means building a stronger belief structure about your life on planet Earth. Your starting point is where you are now. What are your existing beliefs and values? To explore this question, quiet the chatter of your mind and allow your deep thoughts to come to the surface. From a silent mind, consider your beliefs and values. These beliefs and values are the essence of who you are and what you represent. Having well defined beliefs and values means that you have a good structure to control your mind.

Meditation can help you to calm your mind and take control of it. You do not have to go to a class to meditate—just find a quiet place, close your eyes, pay attention to your breathing, and go inside your mind. The goal of meditation is to quiet your thoughts.

Silent observation can assist you to dissolve your ego and become "one with the universe." The Buddhist concept of mindfulness is a good place to start if you want to look for help on the subject of meditation. I consider praying a form of meditation. Yoga is stretching while being mindful of your breathing and this can also be helpful.

Your goal should be to stop the chatter and constant stream of thoughts. Most people can stop their thoughts for only a few seconds, but this can increase if you practice often.

I believe that vibrations connect everything in the universe, so I try to orientate my personal psyche with the concept of "universal consciousness, past, present, and future." I include relatives who have pasted away, my parents, friends, neighbors, and even my family pets as part of my universal consciousness. I include myself and my future self as part of my universal consciousness. This is my "higher power."

I have other beliefs that affect my spiritual health, for example, I believe the Egyptian pyramids were built by intelligent life who found it easy to cut, transport and build with huge blocks of stone. I believe that huge monolithic stone structures and intricate hard-stone carvings found in Egypt, Easter Island, South America, the Middle East and other parts of planet Earth are proof of the existence of intelligent life other than human beings.

I believe that approximately 12,000 years ago, a significant event happened on planet Earth, setting into motion a cascade of events which are poorly explained by our current visions of history.

Many people who have had a near death experience claim that there is a  beautiful parallel universe on the other side of death and there is no reason to be afraid of death. The Western world has largely ignored the subject of death for centuries. There is more research being done today and there is more evidence that physical death is not a return to the "mud" that I once thought it was.

These beliefs give me good spiritual health which promotes my mental well-being and gives me peace of mind. Feeling spiritually centered allows me to manage my day-to-day struggles with more grace and dignity. These ideas have not always been part of my personal belief structure, but they are part of my spirituality today and I find them helpful.

I am not trying to convince you about the merit of my beliefs. I have created my own spiritual beliefs over many years, and I encourage you to do the same. Whatever works for you is fine with me, as long as it does no harm to others. If some of my ideas resonate with you, please use them. If you have ideas of your own, that is even better!

To believe "I do not know" is legitimate position if you are constantly seeking the truth and simply do not have a strong opinion at this time. Live consciously and make decisions for yourself and slowly your spiritual beliefs will become clear to you.

There is no "spiritual police," at least not in America at the time of the writing of this book. No authority is going to arrest you for your spiritual beliefs. You are free to seek a meaningful connection with anything bigger than yourself and this can help you to live with a strong control of your own mind.

**Direction:** Please write down your core beliefs. Start each sentences with "I believe ...".

_____

_____

_____

_____

_____

_____

_____

_____

_____

_____

_____

_____

_____

_____

_____

_____

_____

_____

# 4.6: Improve Your Decision-Making

No one becomes an addict on purpose; children do not dream of growing up to become an addict. Every addict slides into addiction after a long series of poor decisions. Often, these poor decisions are influenced by legitimate trauma or bad luck, but your decision-making is within your control and it must be improved if you are an addict or alcoholic who is going to succeed in recovering from your addiction.

One of the benefits of having a sponsor is that you can review all your decision options with them before you make a decision. Explaining your decision possibilities to your sponsor forces you to consider the options available to you. Get your sponsor's perspective and heed their advice.

Most decisions have some positives (pros) and some negatives (cons). We want the pros to outweigh the cons by 80/20 or more, then the decision is easy. If the decision is 50/50, it is best to wait and make no decision. Do not decide "yes" or "no" on a 50/50 decision. Simply pass on this decision or maintain the status quo in order to make sure you don't make the wrong decision. Don't make a decision if you're not confident about a positive result.

There are three body parts that you can use to make decisions: your head, your gut, and your heart. To use your head, write down all the positives in one column and all the negatives in another column, then analyze which side outweighs the other. The technical name for this is analytical decision-making.

Another way of making decisions is with your "gut," or intuition. The word intuition can be broken down into "inner tuition" or "inner teacher." If you get a "bad gut feeling" about something, don't do it. Sometimes you cannot be specific about your intuition, but you know it when you feel it.

The best body part to make your decisions is your heart. A good time to do this is when you first wake up in the morning. Consider a potential decision and reflect on what feelings and emotions emerge. Reflect on your decision options and be conscious of your feelings evoked by each option. Give yourself the opportunity to realize what your heart is telling you about this decision. Write this information down and give your early morning thoughts a high level of importance because they emerge out of your subconscious mind. The early morning is a good time for you to tune into the feelings of your heart and your emotions around any decision that is buried in your sub-conscious mind.

There are many books written on decision-making techniques. This simple overview is to encourage you to make your decisions thoughtfully, not while you are "asleep at the wheel." It is important to live consciously! Don't absent-mindedly walk into a bar and wonder why you are drunk three hours later. Don't hang out with "friends" who are shooting heroin and wonder why you relapsed again.

Take ownership of your decisions. You have made a series of bad decisions in the past. Now is a good time to improve your decision-making so that you can have a better future.

# 4.7: Improve Your Emotional Quotient

A high emotional quotient (EQ) is displayed when a person does not react strongly to a situation, they do not "freak out," "fly off the handle," or "blow their top" by over-reacting. Having a high emotional quotient is having a mental balance so that you can be flexible and resilient.

Think of a person you know who seems to handle life well—a person who stays calm even when the road of life is bumpy. This person has a high emotional quotient. People who "freak out" all the time have a low emotional quotient.

In your recovery from addiction, it is better to build your emotional quotient as high as possible. Stay calm even when life gets difficult. Emotional quotient can be learned and improved. Read books on this subject and subscribe to YouTube channels that focus on improving your emotional quotient. You will benefit from these efforts by enjoying a smoother day-to-day life. You will be taking control of your mind, which is important for long-term recovery.

# 4.8: Move Toward Your Interests and Fears

The world is constantly changing around you and it is important that you adapt with it. It is necessary to reinvent yourself and keep moving toward the "new and improved" version of yourself.

During the first six months of your sobriety, you have a good opportunity to identify new interests and hobbies you would like to pursue. Since you are not spending all your time getting loaded, there will be a lot of free time and space in your life.

Perhaps you've always wanted to do stand-up comedy, or play a musical instrument, or learn to use a sewing machine, or go surfing. It does not matter what you want to do, it matters that you have some activities you are interested to do. Make a list of three or four activities that interest you, then try all of them. It is likely that one of these activities will capture your interest for the long term, and you will want to keep doing it. These new interests must fit with your self-identity, and they can be replacements for the void that was left after you gave up your addiction.

If you are struggling to find something that interests you, use fear as your guide. If you think of a particular idea or activity and it frightens you a little bit, that is because you have an emotional connection to the idea. I am not talking about ideas that "scare the hell out of you." Don't go swimming with sharks unless you have always wanted to do a cage dive with sharks. Don't go wing-suit flying unless you have always been attracted in this direction. You should slowly and safely expose yourself to activities that scare you just a little bit so that you can work towards learning to control your mind and doing the activity anyway. Confronting your fears in this way will make you a stronger person. Using your fears as a guide will give you valuable insight into identifying new activities and hobbies that will make your life more meaningful for you. Everyone has different fears, and everyone's life is made meaningful in different ways.

Do not spend your time over-analyzing the past. Humans have memory of the past and imagination of the future. Your imagination of fantastic possibilities brings with it the suffering of failed opportunities of the past. Try to have a short memory and focus on your strengths and what you would like to do in the future.

In the long term, most people are driven to create a home and establish a life partner. Your definition of home and life partner should be broad and you should include consideration of both home and life partner in the future that you plan for yourself.

Here are some wise words from Ellen Johnson Sirleaf, the first female Head of State of an African country and the winner of the 2011 Nobel Prize for Peace: "If your dreams don't scare you, they are not big enough."

Once you have gotten through two years of recovery and remained sober, you will have reached the "recovery lifestyle." There is no guarantee that you will be able to maintain sobriety for the rest of your life, so you must keep working on staying sober and maintaining your awareness of the dangers of a relapse.

In the next chapter, I describe what the recovery lifestyle means to me and I ask you to picture what success looks like for you.

**Direction:** Write down your interests and fears.

**Interests:**_____

_____

_____

_____

_____

_____

**Fears:**_____

_____

_____

_____

_____

_____

# Part 5: The Recovery Lifestyle - Picture It

Most addicts who are contemplating the journey of recovery do not need to list the benefits since they already have deep knowledge that their addiction will kill them and others if they don't stop using drugs and alcohol.

The recovery lifestyle involves a better standard of living, more money in your pocket, no hangovers, no dope sickness, less chaos, and less danger. There are numerous benefits to being clean and sober. Understanding these benefits can help you to keep motivated to stay clean and sober when you are struggling with the temptation to go back to your old ways. Temptations will happen. You must remember that struggle is a part of life for everyone.

Managing the stresses and demands of life is difficult for most people. When you are struggling, you are living. Try to celebrate your struggles as a sign of living a full life because "living is struggling" for most people, most of the time. Over time, you can reduce the struggle, but filling your life with soft comforts does not create a meaningful life for most people. Embrace your struggle and enjoy the ride as best you can.

I have listed below the benefits I have experienced from getting clean and sober. Knowing these benefits may be helpful to you to picture what success in long-term sobriety looks like for you?

## 5.1: Consistent Thought Patterns

For me, the biggest benefit to quitting drugs and alcohol has been the increase in the consistency of my thoughts. When I used chemicals to get high, I went back and forth or "flip-flopped" on a subject. My addiction left me confused and generally undecided on almost every subject. I was confused by my addiction and I was confused by my early recovery.

Now that I have been clean and sober for many years, I have consistent thought patterns, I am less undecided and I am less confused. This leaves me feeling more balanced and content. When I go to sleep at night, I think about life in a content state of mind. When I wake up in the morning, I think about life in the same way as when I went to sleep the night before.

When you abuse substances to get "high" above your normal equilibrium, it is followed by a low below your equilibrium, which an addict will often try to override by taking more drugs and alcohol to keep their high. But a crash is inevitable. One of the biggest benefits of being clean and sober is consistently being at your normal equilibrium.

Since I have been clean and sober, I am no longer being pulled all over the place by mood swings and shifting thought patterns. I am "sailing with an even keel" and experiencing life in a consistent manner. This contributes to me feeling content and grateful.

## 5.2: More Meaning

Life is more fun without drugs and alcohol because you don't have to carry the burden of scoring, financing your habit and holding up a fake identity. You become free and liberated from the prison of addiction. Other people see your progress and congratulate you. You will feel good within yourself and your life will be more fun!

If you want to know the meaning of your life, the answer is simple: your life has the meaning you give it.

A life where you contribute to society and are surrounded by people who love you is a life that has more meaning to you and those around you.

If you want a meaningful life, get off drugs and alcohol and stay off them permanently.

## 5.3: More Respect

Recently, I attended the birthday party of a fourteen-year-old boy while I was visiting the Philippines. The boy's father was very proud of his son, so he bought a whole pig to roast for all the guests. The party was a big success until a group of eight men, including the father of the birthday boy, moved away from the party to a table and chairs in the shade away from the sun. They began to pass around a bottle of rum. I knew where things were going, so I turned to leave. But they called me over and said, "Come have a drink with us?" I politely said "No, not today, thank you" and walked away.

Later that day, when the party was over and I was cleaning up, I saw eight empty bottles of rum! Each of the men had consumed approximately one bottle of rum because once you start drinking from another man's bottle, you are expected to buy a bottle to share with the group. The next day, I saw the father of the birthday boy. He looked sick and complained about his headache and upset stomach. It took him two days to recover from that bottle of rum.

I was pleased with how I avoided this situation. I find the company of people who are drinking to be tolerable for their first drink or two, while they are still acting relatively "normal." Once the effect of the alcohol kicks in, their company becomes unbearable for me. Usually the conversation deteriorates into hypothetical speculations and proclamations of love for anyone supporting their wild pontifications. With more alcohol, that love can quickly turn into anger toward anyone who disagrees with them, and any possibility of intellectual conversation will melt like butter in the hot sun.

A month after the pig-roasting birthday party, two of the men who had been drinking together got into a physical fight with each other because one of them believed the other had disrespected him in some way. My experience of the event was positive. Everyone showed me respect and all my interactions with these men have been respectful. If you want other people to have genuine respect for you, do not join them when they are consuming drugs and alcohol.

Set yourself apart from the crowd by recovering from your addiction. People who achieve sobriety gain the respect of their peers, colleagues, and family members. Most people will respect someone who is willing to confront their difficulties, even if they are not successful in overcoming those difficulties. People can see that you are trying and they respect the effort.

## 5.4: More Love

The constant roller coaster of drug abuse makes managing relationships extremely difficult. Family relationships are severely damaged by addiction. Your family may forgive your past behavior, but it is unrealistic to expect them to forget it. However, they will be proud of you and your efforts at recovery. As long as you are sincerely trying to recover from your addiction, you no longer have to deal with the guilt of hurting your family and loved ones.

It is impossible to keep a long-term romantic relationship together if there is heavy alcohol or drug use involved. Alcohol has caused more arguments, fights, and marriage breakups than any other drug. Heavy drug use brings chaos into the life of the user, so a couple using together have little chance of sustaining a meaningful relationship. These relationships are likely to end in chaos, fatigue, incarceration or death.

Having many light, casual relationships is important for a recovering addict. Developing healthy relationships with other people will benefit you, and your life will be more meaningful as a result.

Your path to recovery will lead to less isolation and more healthy social interactions. Over time, your positive relationships are going to help determine the quality of your life. A new relationship will benefit from never having drugs or alcohol involved in it. Getting clean and sober will help in the process of repairing past relationships as well. The more healthy, positive relationships you have, the higher your personal satisfaction with life will be.

Creating a life for yourself that is healthy will attract other people into your life who are also healthy. The best way for you to find a life partner is to be the best version of yourself that you can possibly be and observe who manifests into your life. When other people show interest in you, you should cautiously accept their invitations to connect. Develop your relationships slowly with a series of mutual exchanges of time, effort, and interest. Leading by example, not using drugs or alcohol, you will find other people manifest into your life who are also living a clean and sober lifestyle.

## 5.5: Your Happy Place

Can you think of times and places when you felt happy and content? What are they? Write them down below:

_____

_____

_____

_____

_____

_____

_____

_____

_____

_____

_____

Think of this as your "happy place." Envisioning your happy place gives you some insight into what makes you happy. It gives you a target to aim at. Use your "happy place" as a guiding light even if it is not be possible to get back there because time marches on for all of us. Your happy place may involve people who have passed away, or it may be a time when you were much younger and healthier. Knowing the happy places of your past will give you a good idea of what your happy place of the future looks like.

125

## 5.6: Thrive

Each person in recovery must take care of themself first. Your recovery is of paramount importance and your recovery period is not the time for you to expend a bunch of energy on other people. When you set and pursue your own goals, values, and standards with intent, you will be leading by example and that is the best service you can do for others. Leading by example will have a ripple effect in your community and it will make you attractive to other people.

Determine for yourself what you really want in life and what goals you want to achieve. Be as specific as possible. Write your goals down in your journal. It is never too late to evaluate your life and what matters to you, so now is a good time to start. It will take effort to reach the goals you set, but if you really want them, you will be willing to take on the challenge and willing to put in the effort to achieve them. Once you have set your goals, stop comparing yourself to other people. From now on, only compare yourself to the person you were yesterday and how much closer, or further, you are from your goals.

Being your own person and following your own path is more likely to give you success in recovery and a meaningful life. Always think for yourself and be willing to learn. You will still have to work hard and endure suffering because life is neither easy nor fair for anyone. But if you choose what you want to do, what your values are, and who you want to be, the suffering and hardships you will have to endure can be a pleasurable experience. The purpose of your life is the meaning you give to it. Even your death is more acceptable when you have done what you have wanted to do.

The difference between humans and animals is that humans are conscious being, not compulsive creatures. If your self-imagined drama becomes bigger than your reality in the moment, you can become re-active and feel compelled to act out repeating patterns of behavior which are usually negative. Addicts and alcoholics are prone to repeating patterns of negative behavior. This can bring you to the end of your life in a state of surprise that your life was over so quickly and you did not live the life you wanted to live.

Being your own person and taking control of your life includes choosing your friends and acquaintances. Do not continue to hang out with the people you used to do drugs or alcohol with. Find a new group of friends or "tribe." Your new tribe should be made up of sober people who you respect for different reasons. These people should come from many different backgrounds. If you are going to include a person as a member of your tribe, you should be willing to help this person when they are in need of help. Actively develop your tribe as a group of people that you are proud of.

What most people say should have little bearing on your life. I recommend that you pay little attention to the thoughts and opinions of others; they should not matter to you. What matters is your actions! What you think about is important because it drives your actions. If you are constantly thinking about something, it is likely you will act in that manner sooner or later. Think about positive actions and more importantly, take positive actions. Your actions are what is most important!

I recommend you focus on the actions that you feel give your life purpose and meaning. You are the one who ultimately decides which goals are worthy of your time. This is how you make your own path and be your own person. In the pursuit of the goals you really care about, you will find your happiness.

Lead by example and do not seek the approval of others. This does not mean that you should be rude. Everyone deserves to be treated politely, but you do not need the approval of others. It is important that you become your own person and that you are confident in yourself. Others will be attracted to the energy that you put out, and "miraculously," new people and new opportunities will manifest into your life without you having to forcefully find these people or situations. Good things will come your way because you have set the stage, leading by example and taking positive actions.

Live consciously! Make decisions for yourself and take the actions that you have consciously decided to take. Be your own person and consciously decide for yourself how you will live. This also has a positive impact on all the other people around you who witness you leading by example. You have a ripple effect on your community.

You may be able to re-frame your existing activities to be more focused on helping other people. For example, if you prepare tax returns, you don't think of your job as "filling out forms" but rather re-frame your activity to be people focused and think of your job as "I give people confidence that their tax administration is being efficiently handled." Similarly, if you are a cook, you don't "make meals", you "provide a nutritious solution for people's hunger." If you focus on making other people happy and you will be more happy yourself. This is the "secret" of those who live meaningful lives, filled with love and deep purpose.

Often, our activities outside of our daily work give our lives purpose. If you do activities outside of work for long enough, you may get so good at them that you get paid to do what gives your life meaning. However, this is not possible for everyone. There can be great pleasure and pride in being very good at your job or career, but we are lucky if we get paid to pursue our passions or callings.

Your ultimate goal should be to thrive! What images come to your mind when you image yourself thriving?

**Direction:** Please write below a description of you thriving. Use this description as a target to guide you towards your future.

_____

_____

_____

_____

_____

_____

_____

_____

_____

_____

If you are able to be your own person and thrive within that identity, you will have achieved the goal of taking control of your mind. Thriving will help you to be successful in your long term recovery from addiction and thriving will give you a meaningful life.

What does the "Recovery Lifestyle" mean to you?

**Direction:** Please write down bullet points that describe what your picture of success in recovery from addiction looks like for you?

_____

_____

_____

_____

_____

_____

_____

_____

_____

_____

_____

_____

_____

_131_

# Last Words

Most addicts do not need a list of benefits to motivate them to get clean and sober. You know in your heart that you simply <u>must</u> overcome your addiction. Please allow this book to help you by writing your answers to my questions and writing in the journal pages at the end of this book.

In my story, I shared a scary encounter with a shark. Your addiction is similar to the shark that I faced. It is coming straight at you and it will kill you. Running away from it will make your situation worse. Your best solution is to face it and fight it!

You will have more respect for yourself by facing your problems and trying to overcome them than if you never try. If you try and fail, learn from your mistakes and try again. Setbacks and failures are common in recovery. They happen to most addicts. It is important that you get up and try again.

Quiet the chatter in your mind and live consciously in the moment. You must succeed for a minute, then an hour, then a day—until you have been clean and sober for at least six months. After that, it is likely that you will find staying clean and sober feels easier than it did before and that you no longer need to tell yourself "no" every second, of every day.

Slowly you will transition from saying "no" to your old life to saying "yes" to your new life. Allow your fears and interests to guide you toward activities that give your life meaning. Re-invent yourself as the best version of you that you can be and thrive in your new positive identity.

It was not until I was sober for two years that I realized most of the benefits of being clean and sober. Even after many years of sobriety, no-one is safe from relapse. You must maintain your guard against drugs and alcohol for the rest of your life.

You are not alone. There are many people who are traveling this path with you and there are many people who will help you on your journey. Embrace your struggle and enjoy the ride as best you can.

Feel within yourself that you deeply love yourself and share your love with the people around you! The person who needs your love the most is you!

# Journal

Please use these pages to start your daily journal routine.

Date: _____ Day: _____

What are you grateful for today?

_____
_____
_____
_____

What people did you have positive interactions with today?

_____
_____
_____
_____

What did you do well today?

_____
_____
_____
_____

How did you overcome your cravings today?

_____
_____
_____
_____

Write about your day.

_____
_____
_____
_____
_____
_____

Date: _____ Day: _____

What are you grateful for today?

_____
_____
_____
_____

What people did you have positive interactions with today?

_____
_____
_____
_____

What did you do well today?

_____
_____
_____
_____

How did you overcome your cravings today?

_____
_____
_____
_____

Write about your day.

_____
_____
_____
_____
_____
_____
_____
_____
_____
_____

Date: _____ Day: _____

What are you grateful for today?

_____
_____
_____
_____

What people did you have positive interactions with today?

_____
_____
_____
_____

What did you do well today?

_____
_____
_____
_____

How did you overcome your cravings today?

_____
_____
_____
_____

Write about your day.

_____
_____
_____
_____
_____
_____
_____
_____
_____
_____
_____

Date: _____ Day: _____

What are you grateful for today?

_____
_____
_____
_____

What people did you have positive interactions with today?

_____
_____
_____
_____

What did you do well today?

_____
_____
_____
_____

How did you overcome your cravings today?

_____
_____
_____
_____

Write about your day.

_____
_____
_____
_____
_____
_____
_____
_____
_____
_____
_____

Date: _____ Day: _____

What are you grateful for today?

_____

_____

_____

_____

What people did you have positive interactions with today?

_____

_____

_____

_____

What did you do well today?

_____

_____

_____

_____

How did you overcome your cravings today?

_____

_____

_____

_____

Write about your day.

_____

_____

_____

_____

_____

_____

_____

_____

_____

_____

_____

_____

Date: _____ Day: _____

What are you grateful for today?

_____

_____

_____

_____

What people did you have positive interactions with today?

_____

_____

_____

_____

What did you do well today?

_____

_____

_____

_____

How did you overcome your cravings today?

_____

_____

_____

_____

Write about your day.

_____

_____

_____

_____

_____

_____

_____

_____

_____

_____

_____

Date: _____ Day: _____

What are you grateful for today?

_____
_____
_____
_____

What people did you have positive interactions with today?

_____
_____
_____
_____

What did you do well today?

_____
_____
_____
_____

How did you overcome your cravings today?

_____
_____
_____
_____

Write about your day.

_____
_____
_____
_____
_____
_____
_____
_____
_____
_____
_____

Date: _____ Day: _____

What are you grateful for today?

_____
_____
_____
_____

What people did you have positive interactions with today?

_____
_____
_____
_____

What did you do well today?

_____
_____
_____
_____

How did you overcome your cravings today?

_____
_____
_____
_____

Write about your day.

_____
_____
_____
_____
_____
_____
_____
_____
_____
_____

Date: _____ Day: _____

What are you grateful for today?

_____
_____
_____
_____

What people did you have positive interactions with today?

_____
_____
_____
_____

What did you do well today?

_____
_____
_____
_____

How did you overcome your cravings today?

_____
_____
_____
_____

Write about your day.

_____
_____
_____
_____
_____
_____
_____
_____
_____
_____

Date: _____ Day: _____

What are you grateful for today?

_____
_____
_____
_____

What people did you have positive interactions with today?

_____
_____
_____
_____

What did you do well today?

_____
_____
_____
_____

How did you overcome your cravings today?

_____
_____
_____
_____

Write about your day.

_____
_____
_____
_____
_____
_____
_____
_____
_____
_____

# Epilogue

I have knowledge on the solutions to the problems of
addiction and housing.

Please contact me if you would like to work with me on these subjects.

Thank you.

Paul "Pablo" Noddings

Made in the USA
Monee, IL
29 April 2023

32590721R00090